Hairdressing Science
Second Edition

F. Openshaw, B.Sc., M.I.T.

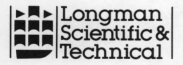

Longman Scientific & Technical
Longman Group UK Limited,
Longman House, Burnt Mill, Harlow
Essex CM20 2JE, England
and Associated Companies throughout the world.

First published 1978
Second impression 1980
Third impression 1982
Fourth impression 1983
Fifth impression 1984
Sixth impression 1985
Second edition 1986
Amended fourth impression 1989
Sixth impression 1993

British Library Cataloguing in Publication Data

Openshaw, Florence
Hairdressing science.—2nd ed.
1. Hairdressing
I. Title
646.7′242′015   TT957
ISBN 0-582-41624-8

Produced by Longman Singapore Publishers Pte Ltd
Printed in Singapore

Contents

Part 1 The hair and head

Part 2 The salon

Part 3 Hairdressing processes

Part 4 Diseases, safety and first aid

Preface to the First Edition

This book is suitable for students studying Hairdressing Science in preparation for the examinations of the City and Guilds of London Institute Hairdressing Certificate (760–01), and those of the Regional Boards.

The traditional method of building up the various stages of science assumes a basic interest by students in that science. This interest is minimal in hairdressing students whose main interest obviously lies with the craft of hairdressing. The book analyses hairdressing topics and introduces sufficient science to explain them. The aim is not only to integrate science with hairdressing but also to integrate the sciences of physics, chemistry and biology together within each topic.

It is hoped that by this approach students may find science easy, interesting and a valuable addition to their knowledge of hairdressing. Pure scientists who are teaching Hairdressing Science for the first time may also find the book a valuable guide in the selection of material.

The questions at the end of each chapter are designed to emphasise and extend important aspects of the work, and provide topics for class discussion. Those at the end of the book will give practice in the type of questions set at City and Guilds' examinations.

I wish to express my gratitude to those who have helped in the preparation of this book, especially Mr Reg O'Brien and Mr John Eaton my former colleagues of Nelson and Colne College, whose criticism and suggestions have been invaluable. I am also deeply indebted to members of my family, particularly my husband, without whose unfailing assistance and advice the work would never have reached print.

Preface to the Second Edition

Although the basic science required for the study of hairdressing science has changed little over the years, hairdressing itself has been constantly developing by the introduction of new products and new equipment. A change of attitude has also taken place, with greater emphasis being placed on good hair condition, and this has led to the use of more acid-based products and to the further development of substantive conditioners. Changes have also taken place in the field of salon services such as in lighting and water heating. Whilst keeping abreast of such developments, the opportunity has been taken to update terminology where appropriate (though of necessity keeping to terms used in the hairdressing and cosmetic industries rather than those exclusive to pure science) and to expand or restructure certain sections of the book. In this way it is hoped that hairdressing students will continue to find the book relevant to modern salon practices.

I gratefully acknowledge the contribution made by former colleagues and friends whose comments and suggestions have again been so valuable and much appreciated.

Foreword

Many hairdressing courses have the subjects of salon practice, science and design taught separately as three distinct areas of work which by some strange alchemy coalesce to form a hairdressing course. Therefore it is often difficult for the young hairdresser to see the relevance of the related subjects to their chosen craft. Usually the science is taught by a pure scientist in a science laboratory which seems far removed from the salon, the client and the work with which the student is familiar or has come to learn.

This book, *Hairdressing Science*, by Florence Openshaw supplies a long-felt need among those concerned with the education and training of hairdressers, to teach science through the student-centred learning approach but also to integrate physics, chemistry and biology with practical hairdressing. Young and aspiring hairdressers will be encouraged on opening the book to see that the first chapters are concerned with the hair and head, the very topics for which they already have an enthusiasm and with which they are familiar. Then come sections on the salon and the processes that take place therein, to be followed by diseases, safety, first aid, and finally examples of multiple choice questions, which are so helpful to the examination candidate.

For a number of years I was fortunate enough to observe the integrated approach to teaching hairdressing science when Florence Openshaw was on the staff of the Nelson and Colne College of Further Education and I was a County Adviser for Further Education with Lancashire. Her success in teaching students by the methods embodied in this book was well proven. In effect, she started with that which they knew, that which was familiar and had an appeal to them as hairdressers. In so doing she was able to teach all the science necessary for the salon operative in a language and terms easily understood and at the same time provide the student with a sufficiently good theoretical and scientific background to confidently tackle the City and Guilds examination papers.

This book will be welcomed by students and lecturers alike as an aid to learning and should do much to remove the dichotomy which often exists between salon and laboratory.

Sheila McIlwrick,
Senior Adviser for Further Education,
Tameside Education Department.

Acknowledgements

The author and publishers would like to thank the following for permission to reproduce photographs in the book:

Britony IIA multipoint water heater manufactured by Chaffoteaux Ltd (Fig. 9.7).

Wella International, Figs. 1.3(*b*); 1.3(*c*); 1.5(*b*).

Dimplex Heating Ltd, Figs. 6.12(*a*); 6.13(*a*).

Eastern Electricity, Harlow, for Fig. 6.14(*a*).

J. A. Crabtree Ltd, Figs. 7.11; 7.14.

Thorn Lighting Ltd, Figs. 8.7; 8.8; 8.14; 8.15.

Houseman Hegro, Permutit Domestic Division, Fig. 9.13; Fig. 9.16(*b*).

Suter Electrical Ltd, Fig. 12.11.

Institute of Dermatology, London, for Figs. 16.5; 16.6.

Part 1
The hair and head

Chapter 1

Hair

Hairdressing is mainly concerned with the care and dressing of the scalp hair, and in the case of men's hairdressing the beard and moustache. This strong coarse hair is known as *terminal hair* but amongst it there is always a smaller amount of soft fine hair or *vellus hair*. Fine downy vellus hair also grows from most parts of the skin except the soles of the feet, palms of the hands and the lips. The hair of the human foetus is even finer, and is known as *lanugo hair*, but this is shed about one month before birth when vellus hair starts to grow. Terminal hair usually replaces the vellus hair of the scalp soon after birth, though many babies are born with a considerable amount of terminal scalp hair. At puberty, terminal hair also replaces vellus hair in the armpits (axillae) and in the pubic area. In males, coarse terminal hair grows at this time in the beard and chest areas as well. If the man later becomes bald, vellus hair is again produced on the scalp in place of terminal hair. Short bristle type hairs grow in the nostrils and also form the eyelashes and eyebrows.

In animals, the main function of hair or fur is to keep the animal warm. In cold conditions the hairs stand erect, trapping an insulating layer of still air in the fur. Birds fluff out their feathers for the same reason. Human body hairs are insufficient for this purpose, though the hairs do stand erect when the body is cold. Scalp hairs help to keep the head warm, cushion it against blows and protect it from damage by ultra-violet rays in sunlight. However, the main purpose of hair is now one of personal adornment. All hairs are sensitive to touch and increase the sensitivity of the skin to light pressure. The presence of bristly hair is usually protective. The eyebrows prevent sweat from running down the forehead into the eyes, whilst the lashes prevent the entry of dust. The nostril hairs filter dust from the air as it is breathed in, so cleaning the air before passage to the lungs.

What is hair?

The part of a hair that is seen above the surface of the skin is the *hair shaft* and, unless the hair has been cut, the tip is always pointed. The hair shaft is composed of a dead, tough horny protein material called *keratin*. The actively growing and therefore living part of the hair is situated below the surface of the skin at the base of a minute pit (about 4 mm deep and 0·4 mm wide) known as a *hair follicle* (see Fig. 1.1). Thus the hair dies as it grows up the follicle, becomes hardened, and emerges from the surface of the skin as a dead material in the form of keratin.

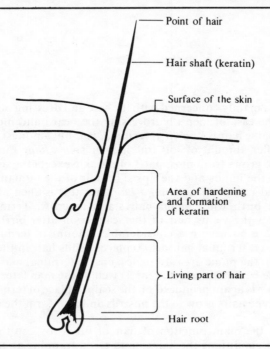

Point of hair

Hair shaft (keratin)

Surface of the skin

Area of hardening and formation of keratin

Living part of hair

Hair root

Fig. 1.1 Section of hair follicle

A closer look at a scalp hair

Experiment 1.1. Examination of a scalp hair
Pull a single hair from your scalp and run your fingers along its length, first in one direction and then in the other direction. You should notice that it feels slightly rougher when you run your fingers towards the end pulled from the scalp. Next, place the hair in a drop of water on a microscope slide, cover with a cover-slip and examine the hair under a microscope. (The surface scales are more easily seen if the hair is previously soaked in glycerol for several hours.)

Microscopic examination of the surface of a hair shows it to be covered with over-lapping scales or imbrications (see Fig. 1.2 and Fig. 1.3b). This outer layer of the hair, the *cuticle*, consists of translucent scales of keratin, with the tips towards the free end or *point of the hair*. The scales fit tightly over each other like the tiles on a roof and tend to prevent water and other liquids from penetrating the hair shaft. They may extend part way round the hair shaft or completely round, to form a ring. The edges of the scales are smooth near the scalp and rougher near the point of the hair.

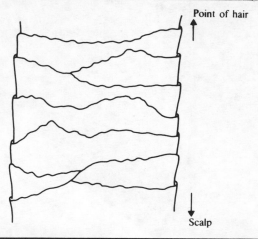

Fig. 1.2 The surface scales of a hair

The thickness of the cuticle depends on the degree of overlapping of the scales (see Fig. 1.3a). In man this varies from 7 to 11 layers. The structure of the cuticle allows the scales to slide over each other when the hair is stretched. This tough outer cuticle serves to hold the whole hair together. The cuticle may be damaged by chemicals or harsh treatment (see Figs. 1.3b and 1.3c).

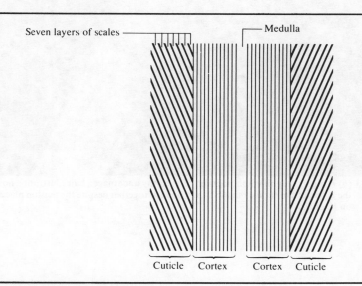

Fig. 1.3 (*a*) Section of hair showing overlapping cuticle scales

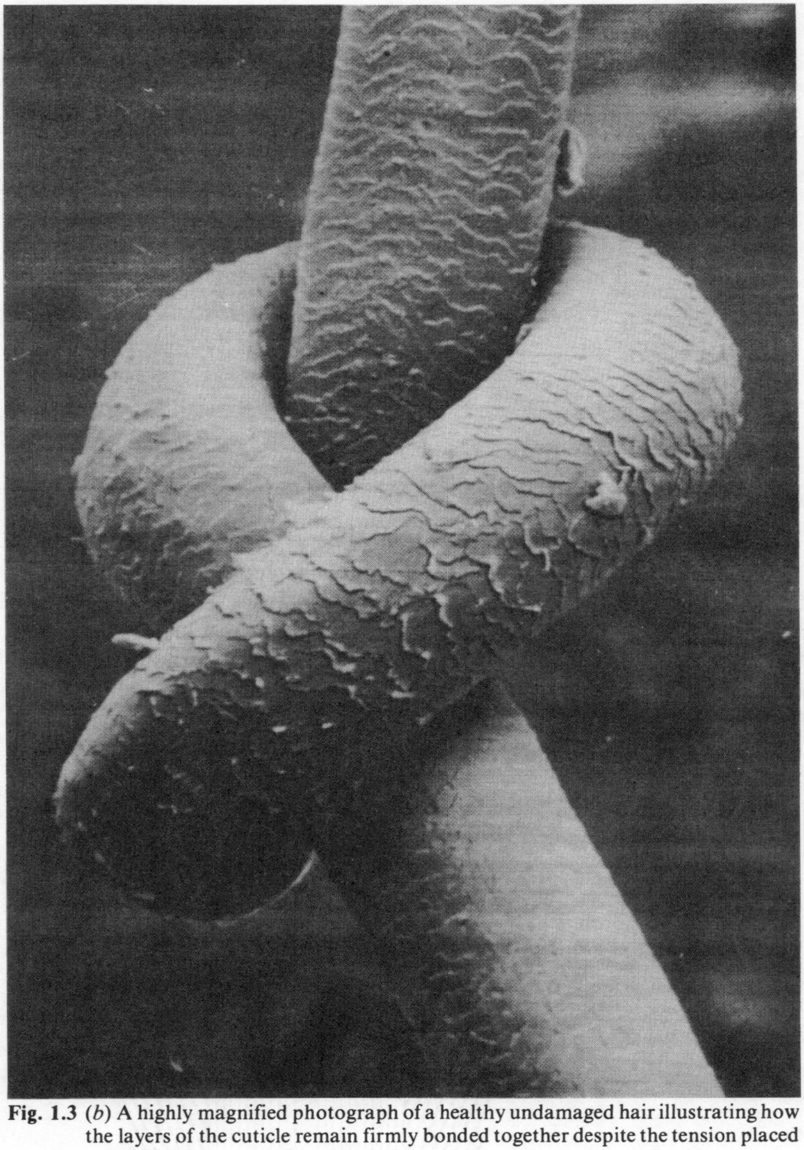

Fig. 1.3 (*b*) A highly magnified photograph of a healthy undamaged hair illustrating how the layers of the cuticle remain firmly bonded together despite the tension placed on the hair.

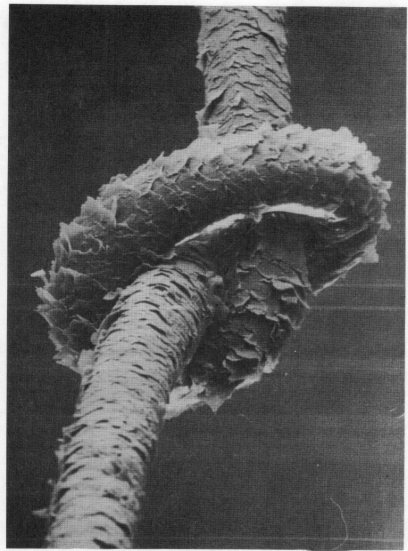

Fig. 1.3 (*c*) A highly magnified photograph of a hair that has been damaged by improper care. It illustrates how the layers of the cuticle have separated and shows how easily this hair would become entangled during styling and thus be harder to work with than healthy undamaged hair.

During the microscopic examination of hair a band called the *medulla* is often seen along the centre of the hair (see Fig. 1.4). This medulla consists of a honeycomb of irregularly shaped areas of keratin with many air spaces between them. The medulla is not present in all scalp hairs, particularly if the hair is fine. Sometimes it is not continuous along the length of the hair. There is no medulla in vellus type hairs.

The main bulk of the hair, between the cuticle and the medulla, is the *cortex*. The elongated cells of this layer contain a tough fibrous type of keratin with long bundles or cables of fibres running parallel to the length of the hair. These are closely bound together by a cementing material or matrix, but there are some air spaces between them. The cortex also contains granules of the pigment *melanin* which is mainly responsible for the colour of the hair.

A hair thus consists of three layers as shown in Fig. 1.4.

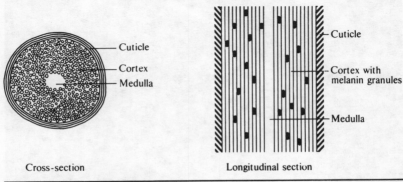

Cross-section   Longitudinal section

Fig. 1.4 Sections of a hair

Looking more closely at the cortex

The cortex is the most important part of the hair for it is this layer which is most affected during various hairdressing processes. During

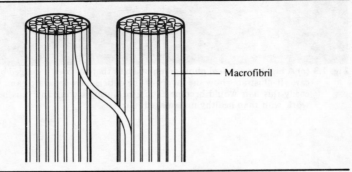

Fig. 1.5 (*a*) The interlocking of protruding fibrils

bleaching, the coloured melanin in the cortex is changed chemically into a colourless substance by the action of hydrogen peroxide. Permanent dyes penetrate into the cortex to add colour to the hair and the chemical structure of the cortex is changed during permanent waving.

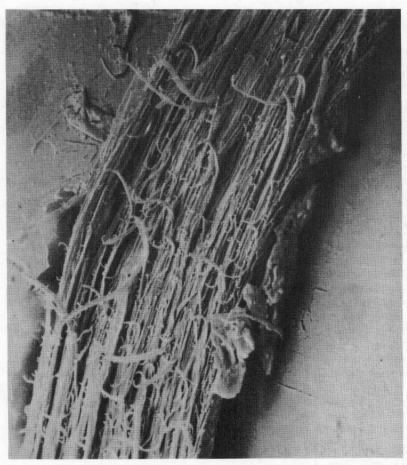

Fig. 1.5 (*b*) A highly magnified photograph illustrating the thread-like inner structure of the cortex of the hair.

By the use of the scanning electron microscope and by X-ray methods, scientists have been able to study the structure of the keratin of the cortex (see Fig. 1.5b). It has been shown to consist of a series of fibres containing even finer fibres. The largest fibres or *macrofibrils*, lying parallel to the length of the hair, are held together by a matrix of twisted keratin fibres and by the interlocking of protruding fibrils (see Fig. 1.5a).

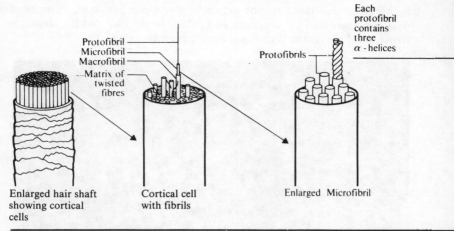

Fig. 1.6 The structure of hair keratin

The macrofibrils are made up of smaller fibres called *microfibrils* which in turn contain *protofibrils*. Each protofibril consists of a group of three coiled chains known as *polypeptide chains*. The chains have a spiral shape called an *alpha-helix* (alpha, written α, is the first letter of the Greek alphabet) and are like minute coiled springs held together by cross linkages in a ladder-like structure (see Fig. 1.6). Since this structure is important in explaining setting and in permanent waving it will be considered again in later chapters. The coils are responsible for the elasticity of hair, enabling it to stretch and to spring back when released.

Boiling hair with hydrochloric acid splits the polypeptide chains into chemical substances called *amino acids* of which there are eighteen different types of keratin. Each amino acid consists of a different arrangement of the *chemical elements* carbon, hydrogen, oxygen and nitrogen chemically united together. Two of the amino acids, cystine and cysteine, also contain the element sulphur in addition to the other four elements mentioned. This is important in the study of perming.

The elements in keratin are present in the following proportion:

Carbon 50 per cent
Oxygen 21 per cent
Nitrogen 18 per cent
Hydrogen 7 per cent
Sulphur 4 per cent

In common with all chemical elements, these substances cannot be split into any simpler substances.

Hair keratin as a chemical substance

The five elements of hair keratin are amongst about a hundred different

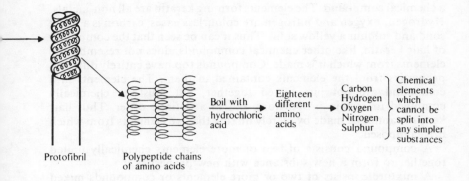

| | Boil with hydrochloric acid | Eighteen different amino acids | Carbon Hydrogen Oxygen Nitrogen Sulphur | Chemical elements which cannot be split into any simpler substances |

Protofibril   Polypeptide chains of amino acids

elements which exist. Elements are the simplest substances obtainable, and may be regarded as the building bricks from which all things, including living organisms, are made. They join together by chemical reaction to form new substances called *compounds*.

Elements

An element is a substance which cannot be split up into any simpler substance. Elements may be divided into two groups, metal elements and non-metal elements. Some of the more important elements are listed in Table 1.1.

Table 1.1 Elements

Metal elements		Non-metal elements			
Aluminium	Lead	Hydrogen		Boron	
Calcium	Magnesium	Chlorine		Carbon	
Copper	Potassium	Fluorine	gases	Phosphorus	solids
Iron	Sodium	Nitrogen		Silicon	
Mercury	Selenium	Oxygen		Sulphur	

Normally *metals* are solids, except mercury, which is a liquid. They have lustre, may be hammered into sheets or drawn into wires, and are good conductors of both heat and electricity. Metals are often attacked by acids forming compounds called salts.

Many *non-metallic elements* are gases. The solid non-metal elements are usually dull and brittle and are poor conductors of heat and electricity. (An exception is carbon in the form of graphite which will conduct an electric current.)

Compounds and mixtures

Because keratin is made up of elements joined together chemically, it is a chemical compound. The elements forming keratin are all non-metals. Hydrogen, oxygen and nitrogen are colourless gases, carbon is a black solid and sulphur a yellow solid. Thus it can be seen that the compound of hair keratin, like other chemical compounds, does not resemble the elements from which it is made. Compounds too have entirely different properties from the elements contained in them. The elements in a compound are not just mixed together, but must be chemically combined in certain proportions and in a definite order. Thus hair keratin cannot be made by merely mixing the five elements from which it is composed.

A compound consists of two or more elements chemically united together to form a new substance with new properties.

A mixture consists of two or more elements or compounds mixed together without being chemically combined. The proportions of the substances in a mixture may be varied and the original substances are usually easily separated, unlike those of a compound. The properties of a mixture are similar to those of the substances from which it is made.

Keratin, like all other proteins, is an *organic compound*, since it contains the element carbon and is obtained from a living organism. Other organic compounds include sugar, alcohol and fat. *Inorganic compounds* have usually a simpler composition than organic compounds and are obtained from non-living sources. Examples are hydrogen peroxide, sulphuric acid, water and ammonia.

Atoms and molecules

The smallest possible particle of an element which can take part in a chemical reaction is *an atom* of that element. The atoms of any one element are all alike, but are different from the atoms of other elements. During chemical reactions atoms join together to form molecules. A *molecule* is defined as two or more atoms chemically united together – or as the smallest part of a substance that can exist by itself.

A molecule of keratin is the smallest part of the compound keratin that exists. Keratin molecules are complex, each containing hundreds of atoms of the elements carbon, hydrogen, oxygen, nitrogen and sulphur arranged in a certain order and present in a fixed proportion.

The properties of hair

1. The colour of hair

This depends on the number and kind of pigment granules in the cortex. The cuticle is translucent so that the colour shows through. Black and brown hairs contain the pigment *melanin*; blonde hairs contain the yellow-red pigment *pheomelanin*; white hairs have little or no pigment; whilst grey hair is considered to be a mixture of white and coloured hairs. Most hairs contain a mixture of pigments.

2. The thickness of hair

Thickness may be measured by using a micrometer screw gauge (see Fig. 1.7), or more accurately, by means of a special attachment to a microscope.

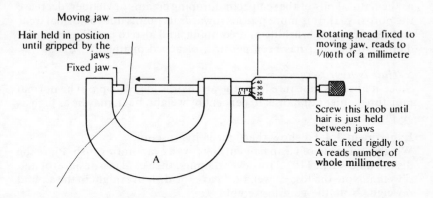

Fig. 1.7 Micrometer screw gauge

A hair is usually the same thickness all along its length and has an average thickness of 0·05 millimetres. If soaked in water, a hair increases in thickness by a greater proportion than it increases in length, as water entering the air spaces between the fibres of the cortex causes the hair to swell.

Experiment 1.2 Comparison of the thickness of hairs
Place a drop of water on a microscope slide. Lay hairs from several different heads across the water and cover it with a cover-slip. Examine the slide under a microscope, and note the differences in colour and variation in thickness of the hairs. Repeat using several hairs from the same head. Cut a single hair into two pieces and soak one piece in water for several hours. Mount both pieces on the same slide and examine for variation in thickness.

3. Hair is elastic

Elasticity is due to the coiled spring structure of keratin and increases if the hair is wet. The stretching of hair is said to be a *physical change* since no chemical reaction takes place and no new substances are formed.

Experiment 1.3 To show the elasticity of hair
Prepare a bundle of about ten hairs each approximately 20 cm long. Knot the hairs together at each end. Soak the bundle in water containing a little shampoo. Holding one end in each hand pull firmly to stretch the hair. The hair may be both felt and seen to stretch, and then to spring back when released.

4. Hair is porous

Liquids pass between the cuticle scales into the cortex, the porosity depending on the state of the cuticle. If the cuticle has been damaged or if the scales have been lifted by treatment with dry heat, steam or alkalis, the porosity is increased. Substances coating the hair shaft, such as the natural oils of the scalp, conditioning creams or lacquer, decrease the porosity. Hair is more porous towards its points due to normal wear and tear through brushing and combing, and also to possible chemical damage if the hair has been permed, bleached or tinted.

5. Hair is hygroscopic

Since it absorbs moisture from the air, hair is hygroscopic. The normal moisture content of hair is 10 per cent by weight, but it may be as high as 30 per cent.

Experiment 1.4 To show that hair is hygroscopic
Weigh a quantity of clean hair cuttings in an evaporating dish. Place the dish in an oven at 110°C for several hours, then cool in a desiccator and reweigh. Note the loss of weight. Leave the dish overnight in the air and reweigh. Note the gain in weight.

6. The texture or 'feel' of hair

A combination of some of the properties already mentioned determines the texture of hair which depends on:
(a) the thickness of the hair;
(b) the degree of roughness of the cuticle;
(c) the moisture level of the cortex;
(d) the length of the hair. Very short hair seems stiff, whilst long hair seems softer.

7. The action of acids and alkalis on hair

Hair reacts differently to the two groups of chemical substances known as *acids* and *alkalis*, and their identification in hairdressing preparations is therefore important. The presence of acids and alkalis may be

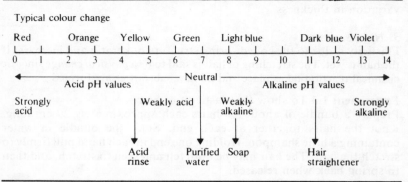

Fig. 1.8 The pH scale

detected by the change in colour of an *indicator paper* impregnated with *litmus* dye. Red litmus paper turns blue in alkaline liquids and blue litmus paper turns red in acids. The use of *universal* indicator paper (pH paper) however not only shows the presence of acids or alkalis, but also indicates the strength of the acid or alkali by changing through a wide range of colours corresponding to a numerical pH scale of 0 to 14 (see Fig. 1.8). Values below 7 indicate acidity (the lower the number the *stronger* the acid), whilst values of 7 to 14 indicate increasing alkalinity. A substance which is neither acid nor alkaline is *neutral* and has a pH of 7.

Acids may be divided into two groups:
(a) *Inorganic or mineral acids* such as sulphuric acid, hydrochloric acid and phosphoric acid. These are strong acids used in the laboratory and in the manufacture of other chemical compounds such as soapless detergents. Strong acids with a pH of 1–2 will burn the skin and damage cotton fabrics. They make hair feel harsh and stringy, but do not destroy it unless the hair is boiled with the acid. They are not used by themselves in the salon or on hair.
(b) *Organic acids* such as citric acid (found in lemon juice), acetic acid (in vinegar) and tartaric acid (in grapes). These are weak acids and dilute solutions may be used directly on the hair. Weak acids with a pH of 5–6 will condition hair by closing the cuticle scales so making the hair feel smoother (see Fig. 1.9).

Alkalis such as ammonium hydroxide, sodium hydroxide and potassium hydroxide are used in some hairdressing processes although, in general, they are more damaging to hair than are acids. Alkalis feel soapy to the touch, have a bitter taste and attack woollen fabrics. Sodium hydroxide (caustic soda) and potassium hydroxide (caustic potash) are known as *caustic alkalis*. They will burn the skin and destroy hair unless very dilute. Strong alkalis with a pH value greater than 9·5 destroy hair by attacking the polypeptide chains. The hair is softened until it becomes jelly-like and finally disintegrates. Thus they would act as a depilatory or hair remover if applied to the skin or scalp. Weakly alkaline solutions with a pH of less than 9·5, such as soap solutions and dilute ammonium hydroxide, make hair swell and will roughen the hair cuticle (see Fig. 1.9).

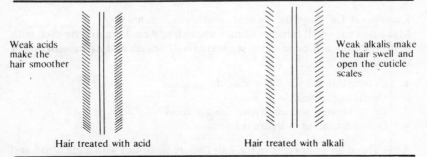

Weak acids make the hair smoother

Hair treated with acid

Weak alkalis make the hair swell and open the cuticle scales

Hair treated with alkali

Fig. 1.9 The effect of acids and alkalis on hair

Although alkalis roughen the cuticle and may cause hair damage, many hairdressing preparations are made alkaline deliberately during manufacture. Ammonium hydroxide is often added to make the hair swell, so allowing the easy entry of other substances such as perm lotions, bleaches and dyes into the hair shafts. Processes involving alkaline substances are often followed by rinses with dilute acids (acetic acid or citric acid) to neutralise any alkali left on the hair and to return the hair to a slightly acid state. The chemical reaction between an acid and an alkali is called *neutralisation* and results in the formation of a salt and water. New substances are always formed during a chemical change and the reaction may be represented by an equation. Neutralisation may be represented as follows:

$$\text{An acid} + \text{an alkali} = \text{a salt} + \text{water}$$

Many different salts may be formed by the process of neutralisation or by the action of acids on metals. A *salt* always consists of a metal or ammonium radical (from the alkali) and an acid radical (from the acid). Thus ammonium thioglycollate (used in perm lotion) is a salt formed by the chemical reaction between thioglycollic acid and ammonium hydroxide; sodium stearate (a soap) is the salt of stearic acid and sodium hydroxide; sodium chloride (common salt) is the salt of hydrochloric acid and sodium hydroxide. Salts are usually neutral with a pH of 7 and have little effect on hair condition. A few, such as soap, borax and sodium carbonate (washing soda), are alkaline and if used on hair tend to roughen the cuticle scales and make the hair swell.

Experiment 1.5 Testing substances for acidity and alkalinity
Using a small quantity of each substance in a separate test tube, test various liquids used in hairdressing first with litmus paper and then with pH paper. Include soap and soapless shampoos, perm lotions, setting lotions, lacquers and conditioners. Also test various laboratory reagents including some of the acids and alkalis mentioned above. Make a pH chart as shown in Fig. 1.8, and place the substance tested on the scale. What effect will each substance have on hair?

Experiment 1.6 The effect of acids and alkalis on hair.
Make up four small bundles of hair about 6 to 8 cm long and tie each with cotton. Place each bundle in a separate small beaker and cover with one of the following:

1.   Concentrated hydrochloric acid.
2.   Dilute acetic acid.
3.   Concentrated sodium hydroxide solution.
4.   Dilute ammonium hydroxide.

After about an hour remove the hair (where possible) with a glass rod and transfer to a beaker of water. Rinse the hair thoroughly with cold water.

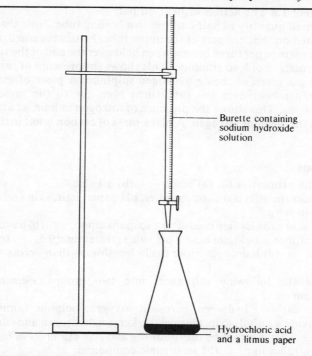

Burette containing
sodium hydroxide
solution

Hydrochloric acid
and a litmus paper

Fig. 1.10 Neutralisation

Compare the 'feel' and strength of the fibres, first whilst wet and then when dry.

N.B. Care must be taken, since both strong acids and strong alkalis burn the skin.

Experiment 1.7 Neutralisation (see Fig. 1.10)
Place 25 ml of dilute hydrochloric acid in a conical flask and add a piece of litmus paper. Gradually add dilute sodium hydroxide solution (an alkali) from a burette until the red litmus paper just begins to turn blue. The solution is then neutral. The salt (sodium chloride in this case) is left behind if the water is boiled away.

Hydrochloric acid + sodium hydroxide = sodium chloride + water
     (acid)   (alkali)   (salt)

8. The action of heat on hair
When hair is heated by dry heat, the cuticle scales are raised and moisture is lost from the hair cortex. Strong heating results in the chemical decomposition of hair, leaving a black mass of carbon. The out-dated practice of singeing the ends of hair by a flame often resulted in globules of carbon left at the free ends of the hair shafts.

Experiment 1.8 The action of heat on hair
Heat a small quantity of hair cuttings in a boiling tube. Note that water
is deposited on the cool part of the upper tube. Notice the smell. A piece
of lead acetate paper turns brown when held over the end of the tube due
to the formation of lead sulphide. This shows the presence of sulphur in
hair, the gas given off being hydrogen sulphide. A piece of moist red
litmus paper held over the tube turns blue due to the presence of
ammonia gas. This shows the presence of nitrogen in hair, as ammonia
contains the element nitrogen. A black mass of carbon is left in the tube.

Questions

1. List the properties of: (a) acids   (b) alkalis.
   Consider the effects on litmus paper, pH paper, hair, skin and metals.
2. Explain why:
   (a) an acid rinse is often used after a soap shampoo;   (b) hairdressing
   preparations should not have a pH value greater than 9·5;   (c) hair is
   elastic;   (d) hairs split more easily lengthways than across the hair
   shaft.
3. Divide the following substances into two groups, elements and
   compounds:
   water, carbon, hydrogen peroxide, oxygen, sulphur, ammonium
   hydroxide, alcohol, soap, aluminium, keratin, hydrogen and citric acid.
4. Explain what is meant by the following and give examples in each case:
   (a) neutralisation;   (b) an organic compound;
   (c) a depilatory;   (d) a hygroscopic substance.
5. Classify the following into physical and chemical changes:
   (a) the swelling of hair when soaked in water;   (b) the action of
   strong heat on hair;   (c) the neutralisation of an alkali on the hair, by
   using an acid rinse;   (d) the stretching of a hair.

Chapter 2

The growth of hair

Hair, like all living material, grows by the division of cells. Each cell is a microscopic unit of living matter consisting of a jelly-like mass, the cytoplasm, surrounded by a membrane through which nourishment can pass into the cell, and through which waste products can leave the cell. A nucleus, usually at the centre of the cell, controls its activity. Groups of cells form tissues such as skin tissue and nerve tissue.

Experiment 2.1. The examination of cells
A sample of cells may easily be obtained by scraping the inside of the cheek with a clean spoon or spatula. Place the sample in a drop of water on a slide and cover. Irrigate with iodine by drawing a drop of iodine solution under the cover-slip using blotting paper. Examination under a microscope shows flat pavement cells which form a smooth lining for the cheek (see Fig. 2.1).

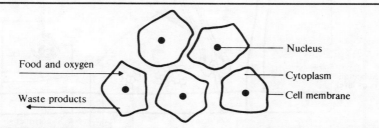

Fig. 2.1 Cell structure

New cells are produced in various parts of the body when one cell splits into two parts (see Fig. 2.2). The nucleus divides first, followed by the cytoplasm.

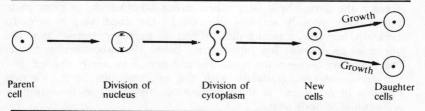

Fig. 2.2 Cell division

The division of cells at the base of the hair follicles in the skin produces the new cells required for hair growth. In order to understand this growth it is necessary to study the structure of the skin and the hair follicles themselves.

The structure of the skin

The skin consists of two main layers:
1. **The epidermis** or outer layer.
2. **The dermis** or true skin forming the inner layer (see Fig. 2.3).

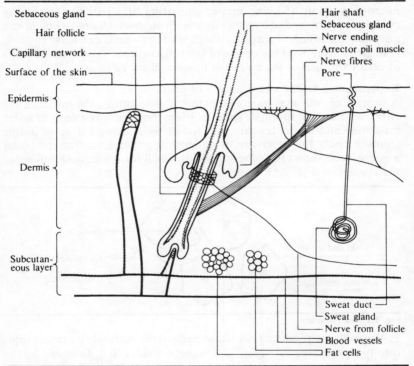

Fig. 2.3 Section through the skin

Beneath the dermis is a fatty *subcutaneous layer* which, in most parts of the body, loosely attaches the skin to the underlying muscle. In the scalp, however, a strong sheet of fibrous tissue or tendon called the *epicranial aponeurosis* lies immediately below the subcutaneous tissue. The boundary between the epidermis and dermis is clearly defined, but the dermis merges gradually with the subcutaneous layer. Varying amounts of fat stored in the subcutaneous tissue act as insulation to prevent loss of body heat.

The surface of the skin and hair is coated with the slightly acid secretions of two types of gland:

1. **Sebaceous glands** open into the hair follicles and secrete an oily substance called sebum which lubricates the skin and hair shafts so helping to make them waterproof. Sebum gives lustre to the hair, though excess makes the hair greasy.

2. **Sweat glands** are coiled tubes lying in the dermis with a duct leading to an opening or pore on the surface of the skin. Sweat consists of about 98 per cent water and 2 per cent sodium chloride (common salt) with traces of many other substances. The liquid sweat takes heat from the skin when it evaporates and this cools the body.

The epidermis

The epidermis consists of several layers of cells, constantly changing from an actively growing lower layer to an upper layer of dead scale-like cells which are gradually rubbed away by friction and are replaced from below. The outer layer consists mainly of flaky scales of the tough protein keratin, which forms a waterproof coat for the body and protects the underlying tissue from infection, dirt and injury. It also prevents excessive loss of water from the body tissues. There are very few nerves in the epidermis and no blood vessels. The lower living layer is nourished by blood vessels in the dermis. The thickness of the epidermis varies from about 0·1 mm to 2 mm in different parts of the body, being thin in the eyelids and abdomen, and thickest on the soles of the feet and palms of the hands.

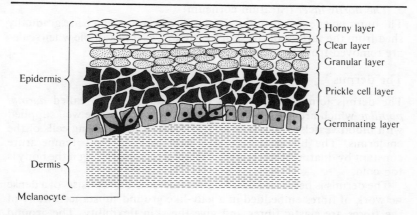

Fig. 2.4 The structure of the epidermis

The layers of the epidermis are shown in Fig. 2.4. Starting with the lowest layer, they are as follows:

1. The germinating layer or basal layer   (Stratum germinativum)
This actively growing layer consists of regularly arranged cells which are constantly dividing to form new cells, so pushing the old cells

towards the surface of the skin. The germinating layer is continuous round the hair follicles, sebaceous glands and sweat glands, and although these structures may appear to be part of the dermis, they are all down growths of the epidermis. Amongst the cells of this layer are smaller cells called *melanocytes*, which produce the pigment of the skin in the form of yellow, brown or black granules of melanin. Sunbathing increases the production of melanin which protects the skin from damage by the sun's rays, the dark pigment absorbing harmful radiations.

2. The prickle cell layer (Stratum spinosum)
This is also known as the Stratum aculeatum. Some of the soft, nucleated cells of this layer have a spiny outgrowth through which it is thought that melanin granules enter the cells. Together with the germinating layer, it forms the living part of the epidermis or *Malpighian layer.*

3. The granular layer (Stratum granulosum)
The nuclei of the cells in this layer are breaking down, leading to the death of the cells. Keratin is being formed in the cells.

4. The clear layer (Stratum lucidum)
The flattened cells of this layer contain keratin and have no nuclei. Melanin granules are destroyed in the cells.

5. The horny layer (Stratum corneum)
The outer layer consists of flat dead cells of keratin which are gradually shed from the surface of the skin by friction, as for example when scales are removed from the scalp during brushing.

The dermis

The dermis joins the epidermis in a series of ridges called *dermal papillae* which are shallow in the scalp. The papillae are well supplied with blood vessels which take nourishment to the growing cells of the epidermis. The blood vessels also help to keep body temperature constant by dilating if the body is too hot and constricting if the body is too cold.

The dermis is between 1 and 4 mm in thickness and consists of a dense network of fibres embedded in a jelly-like ground substance. Many of the fibres are elastic fibres and give the skin flexibility. The ground substance holds a lot of water which makes the skin turgid (firm).

Nerve endings of several types are found in the dermis making the skin sensitive to pain, heat, cold and pressure. These sensations are carried along nerves to the brain.

The structure of a hair follicle

A hair follicle (see Fig. 2.5) is formed by the downgrowth of the epidermis into the dermis, the outside of the follicle being a continuation of the germinating layer of the epidermis. The walls of the follicle are known as the *outer root sheath*. The dermis forms a protective sheath of connective tissue round each follicle and also projects upwards into the base of the follicle forming the *hair papilla*. The hair grows from the epidermal cells surrounding the papilla, the cells being nourished from the blood vessels which enter the papilla.

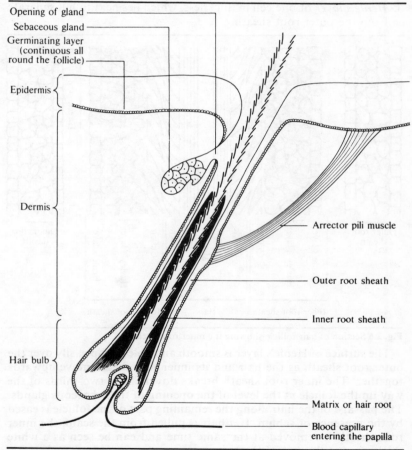

Fig. 2.5 The structure of a hair follicle

A small muscle, the *arrector pili muscle*, is attached to each hair follicle. Cold conditions or fear cause this muscle to contract, moving the sloping follicle and making the hair stand erect, and also making the skin rise in a goose-pimple. The erection of the hair is an attempt by the body to trap an insulating layer of still air between the hairs and skin to prevent heat loss by the body. It is ineffective in man due to lack of body hair.

Whilst in the follicle, the hair itself is surrounded and protected by the *inner root sheath* which grows up along side the hair. The inner root sheath consists of three layers (see Fig. 2.6).

1. *A cuticle* with overlapping scales pointing to the base of the follicle and so interlocking with the cuticle of the hair and holding the hair firmly.
2. *Huxley's layer* of 2 or 3 cells thickness.
3. *Henle's layer* of one cell in thickness, which lies next to but separate from the outer root sheath.

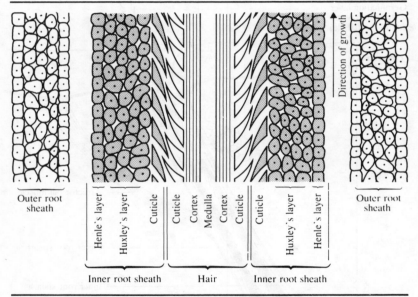

Fig. 2.6 Section of hair follicle showing the inner root sheath

The surface of Henle's layer is smooth and able to slip easily over the outer root sheath as the hair and its inner root sheath move upwards together. The inner root sheath breaks down about two-thirds of the way up the follicle at the level of the opening of the sebaceous glands. The passage of the hair along the remaining part of the follicle is eased by the presence of sebum. If a hair is pulled from the scalp, the inner root sheath is removed at the same time and can be seen as a white thickening at the end of the hair.

The growth cycle of a hair

The lower part of the follicle widens out into the *hair bulb* (see Fig. 2.7), which fits over the hair papilla. The epidermal cells surrounding the papilla form the *germinal matrix* or root of the hair. These cells are constantly dividing to make new cells which push the older ones upwards. At first all the cells are alike but as they move up the follicle they begin to change shape, and keratin develops in the cells. The different types of cell for the cuticle, cortex and medulla of the hair and the cells of the inner root sheath develop. By the time they are about one-third of the way up the follicle the cells are dead and fully keratinised. Between the cells surrounding the papilla are melanocytes producing melanin, the pigment of the hair, most of which passes into the cortex of the hair.

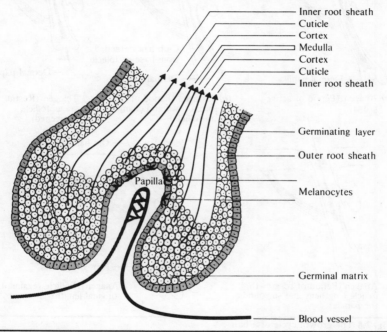

Inner root sheath
Cuticle
Cortex
Medulla
Cortex
Cuticle
Inner root sheath

Germinating layer

Outer root sheath

Melanocytes

Papilla

Germinal matrix

Blood vessel

Fig. 2.7 The hair bulb

A scalp hair continues to grow for between two and seven years, growing at a rate of about 1·25 cm per month. Thus the final length, if never cut, would vary from about 30 to 100 cm. During the period of active growth the follicle is said to be in *anagen* (see Fig. 2.8).

At the end of the growth period changes occur in the follicle. The hair stops growing and becomes detached from the base of the follicle forming a *club hair*. The hair bulb begins to break down and the follicle becomes shorter. A narrow section of the outer root sheath remains in contact with a group of cells which formed the hair papilla. During this period of change the follicle is in *catagen*, a phase which lasts for about two weeks.

The follicle then enters a resting stage known as *telogen* for three to four months. After this time the follicle lengthens again and a new bulb develops round the cells of the original papilla. A new hair starts to grow when the follicle has reached its full length. If the old hair is still in the follicle, it is pushed out by the new growth.

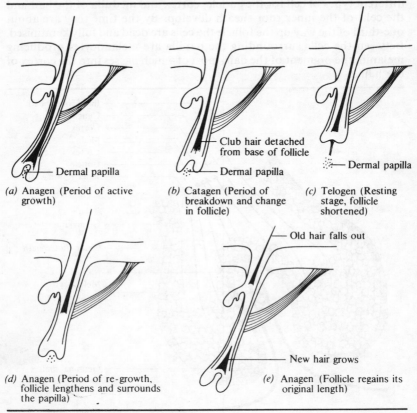

(a) Anagen (Period of active growth)

(b) Catagen (Period of breakdown and change in follicle)
— Club hair detached from base of follicle
— Dermal papilla

(c) Telogen (Resting stage, follicle shortened)
— Dermal papilla

— Dermal papilla

(d) Anagen (Period of re-growth, follicle lengthens and surrounds the papilla)

(e) Anagen (Follicle regains its original length)
— Old hair falls out
— New hair grows

Fig. 2.8 The growth cycle of a hair

In some animals many follicles enter the resting stage at the same time and the animal moults. In humans, the follicles are at different stages in the growth cycle so there is a small but constant shedding of about a hundred scalp hairs per day. This also accounts for the uneven growth of scalp hair and the need for regular cutting.

Factors affecting hair growth

Hair grows more slowly during illness and increased hair loss may follow feverish illnesses, severe shock and the use of various drugs.

The growth of hair is also affected by diet. This is most obvious in some developing countries where the diets of young children are often seriously lacking in protein. The first sign of this protein deficiency is a change in hair colour. Normally black hair becomes red due to a reduction in the amount of melanin produced. The hair may eventually lose all its colour and become very thin and easily broken due to a reduction in keratin formation. These are the symptoms of a condition known as *kwashiorkor*.

Hair tends to grow more quickly in children than in adults, and growth is even slower in old age. It is slightly faster in women than in men. Ultra-violet rays in sunlight speed cell division so that hair grows faster in the summer months. Cutting and shaving have no effect on the rate of hair growth.

Hormones, the secretions from certain glands, also affect hair growth. Lack of hormone secretion from the thyroid gland results in the growth of poor, thin hair. Changes in hormone level in pregnancy and by taking contraceptive pills may also slow hair growth.

Questions

1. Draw a diagram to show a cross section of a hair follicle.
2. What is meant by each of the following:
   (a) kwashiorkor;   (b) evaporation;   (c) a club hair;
   (d) an insulator of heat;   (e) the secretion of a gland.
3. What are the functions of the skin?
4. What is the function of each of the following:
   (a) the inner root sheath;   (b) sebum;   (c) sweat;
   (d) the arrector pili muscle; (e) the stratum germinativum;
   (f) melanin in the skin.
5. Explain why:
   (a) some people find it impossible to grow their hair longer than shoulder length, whilst others are able to grow it much longer;
   (b) hair grows unevenly after trimming.

Chapter 3

The nutrition of the growing hair

The growth of hair depends on the constant division of the cells surrounding the hair papillae. The newly formed cells must then change in shape and become keratinised as they travel along the hair follicles. The materials required for the growth and development of hair are brought to the hair papillae by the blood. These materials include the products of the digestion of the food we eat, and oxygen from the air we breathe in. Thus the nourishment of hair involves the digestive system, the respiratory system and the blood system.

Materials required for the nourishment of hair

The dividing cells in the germinal matrix require a supply of *energy* to enable various chemical reactions to take place inside the cells. Energy is produced when oxygen from the air breathed in reacts chemically with glucose. The chemical reaction is an *oxidation process* since it involves the addition of oxygen to the glucose.

Glucose + oxygen = carbon dioxide + water + energy

Glucose is a type of sugar obtained mainly from the digestion of carbohydrate foods (starches and sugars) but may also be obtained by the breakdown of fats or from any amino acids not required for building new cells. The oxidation of glucose would take place very slowly if vitamins of the B group were not present. These vitamins act as *catalysts*, which are substances that speed up a chemical reaction without being changed themselves.

Other vitamins and minerals also play a part in the growth of hair. Vitamin C is necessary to make the cementing material between cells, and vitamin A affects the formation of keratin. The mineral element iron is required to form the red blood cells which carry oxygen in the blood.

Mature hair consists mainly of the protein keratin which, like other proteins, is built up from smaller units called amino acids. During digestion, protein foods such as eggs, meat, fish and milk are broken down into amino acids. These are circulated in the blood stream, sorted and rearranged to be built up into keratin in the cells of the hair.

Protein in food $\xrightarrow{\text{digested}}$ amino acids $\xrightarrow[\text{in hair cells}]{\text{built up}}$ keratin (protein in hair)

The nutrition of hair thus depends on the nutrients supplied by the digestion of food and on the intake of oxygen from the air. The various nutrients in food with their uses and sources are listed in Table 3.1.

Table 3.1 The sources and uses of nutrients

Nutrient	Foods providing a good source	Use in the body	Result of deficiency in the diet
Protein	Eggs, meat, fish, milk, cheese (animal proteins) Peas, beans, soya beans, nuts, (vegetable proteins)	Building new cells, e.g. new hair, nails and skin cells. May also produce energy	Little danger of lack in U.K. diets Kwashiorkor: stunted growth, blotchy skin, poor, thin hair, loss of hair colour
Carbohydrate 1. starches 2. sugars	Potatoes, bread, cereals Sugar, syrup, jam	To provide energy	Little danger except in starvation conditions
Fats	Butter, cream, cheese	To provide energy Storage in skin provides insulation	Diet less satisfying; feel hungry soon after a meal
Mineral elements 1. Calcium 2. Iron	Milk, cheese Liver, egg-yolk, green vegetables	To build strong teeth and bone To build haemo-globin for red blood cells which carry oxygen in the blood stream	Rickets Anaemia (lack of red blood cells)
Vitamins Vitamin A (retinol)	Dairy produce, margarine, liver, carrots Fish-liver oils Fatty fish	Vital for the correct functioning of the retina in the eyes. Prevents keratin from forming in the lining of the nose and throat and on the front of eyeballs	Night-blindness Dry nose and throat leading to infection Keratin plugs in follicles of upper arms and legs Blindness
Group B vitamins	Cereals, meat, liver	Release of energy from carbohydrates	Affects nerves, skin and digestion of food
Vitamin C (Ascorbic acid)	Oranges, black-currants Green vegetables	To build the cementing material between cells Helps with the absorption of iron	Scurvy. Sore gums, loose teeth, easy bruising. Poor healing of wounds
Vitamin D (Calciferol)	Dairy foods (also made in skin by the action of sunlight)	To ensure the building of strong teeth and bones	Rickets

The digestion and absorption of food

Digestion is necessary to break down food into simple substances which can be absorbed into the blood stream. The alimentary canal, in which digestion takes place, is a continuous tube starting at the mouth and finishing at the anus (see Fig. 3.1). Various substances enter the alimentary canal from the salivary glands, the liver and pancreas to aid digestion. Food is first broken down mechanically by the teeth during chewing and then by the churning movement of the stomach. The main breakdown however is by chemical action brought about by organic catalysts or *enzymes* secreted by the walls of the digestive tract itself, or by glands such as the salivary glands and the pancreas. Each digestive enzyme will only act on one kind of nutrient. Some enzymes like the amylase in saliva work best in alkaline conditions, and others such as the protease in the stomach in acid conditions. The stages of digestion for each nutrient, and the end products of their digestion are shown in Table 3.2. Vitamins and minerals do not require digestion and are absorbed unchanged.

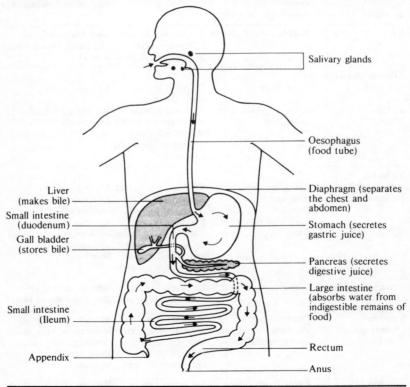

Fig. 3.1 The digestive system

Table 3.2 Digestion

Nutrient	Place of digestion	Digestive juice	Enzyme	Chemical reaction	Product of digestion
Protein	Stomach	Gastric juice	Protease (pepsin)	Protein————>peptones	
	Small intestine (duodenum)	Pancreatic juice	Protease (trypsin)	Peptones————>polypeptides	Amino acids
	Small intestine (ileum)	Intestinal juice	Protease (erepsin)	Polypeptides————>amino acids	
Carbohydrates (starches and sugars)	Mouth	Saliva	Salivary amylase	Cooked starch————>maltose	
	Small intestine (duodenum)	Pancreatic juice	Pancreatic amylase	Starch————>maltose	Glucose
	Small intestine (ileum)	Intestinal juice	Maltase Sucrase	Maltose————>glucose Sucrose————>glucose	
Fats	Small intestine (duodenum)	Bile (an emulsifier not a digestive juice)	—	No chemical action Breaks fat up into small droplets (an emulsion)	Fatty acids and glycerol
	Small intestine (duodenum)	Pancreatic juice	Lipase	Fats————>fatty acids and glycerol	

Digestion begins in the mouth, continues in the stomach and the small intestine, and is completed in the ileum or lower part of the small intestine. The digested food is then absorbed through the walls of the ileum and enters fine blood vessels which surround the ileum wall. The absorbed products of digestion pass along the portal vein to the liver and then travel to the heart which circulates them through the blood to all parts of the body (see Fig. 3.2). The indigestible part of food passes into the large intestine where water is absorbed. The remainder is passed out of the body through the anus.

How oxygen reaches the blood stream

Oxygen needed to oxidise glucose in the body cells is obtained from the air during breathing. This rhythmic process normally takes place about sixteen to seventeen times a minute. Air is forced through the air passages in the head (see Fig. 3.3), and so into the lungs (see Fig. 3.4), by atmospheric pressure when the chest increases in volume. This increase is brought about by the lowering of the diaphragm due to the contraction of the diaphragm muscles, and by the upwards and outwards movement of the ribs due to contraction of the intercostal muscles between the ribs (see Fig. 3.5).

The air in the lungs is forced out of the body, when the volume of the chest decreases due to the relaxation of the diaphragm muscles, so

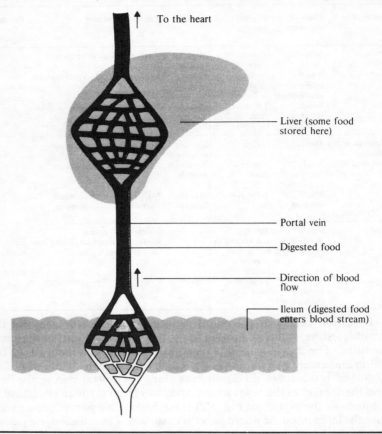

To the heart

Liver (some food stored here)

Portal vein

Digested food

Direction of blood flow

Ileum (digested food enters blood stream)

Fig. 3.2 Digested food enters the blood system

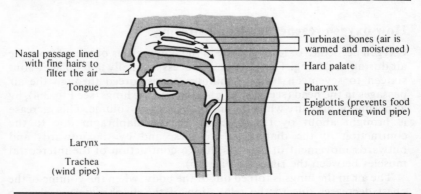

Turbinate bones (air is warmed and moistened)

Nasal passage lined with fine hairs to filter the air

Hard palate

Tongue

Pharynx

Epiglottis (prevents food from entering wind pipe)

Larynx

Trachea (wind pipe)

Fig. 3.3 The air passages in the head

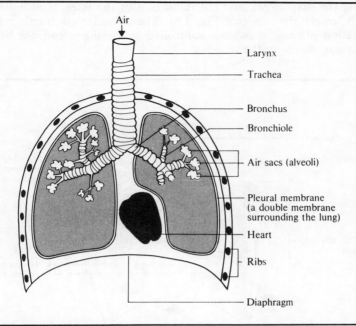

Fig. 3.4 Air passages in the chest

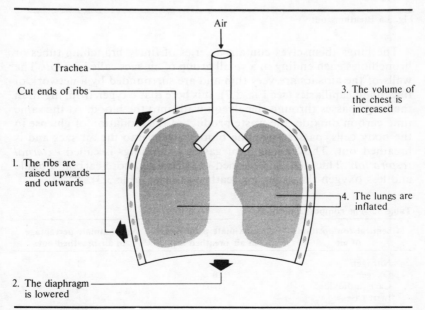

Fig. 3.5 Breathing in

raising the diaphragm, and the relaxation of the intercostal muscles which lowers the ribs (see Fig. 3.6). The alternate contraction and relaxation of these muscles is controlled by messages from the brain sent along nerves to the muscles.

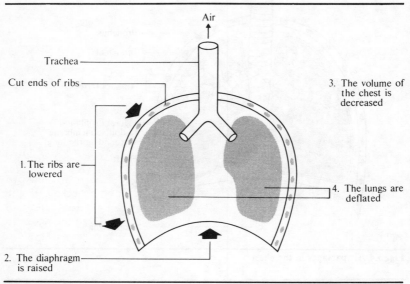

Air

Trachea

Cut ends of ribs

3. The volume of the chest is decreased

1. The ribs are lowered

4. The lungs are deflated

2. The diaphragm is raised

Fig. 3.6 Breathing out

The lungs themselves contain a series of finely branching tubes or bronchioles each ending in a small group of air sacs called *alveoli*. The walls of the air sacs are very thin and are surrounded by a network of fine blood capillaries (see Fig. 3.7). It is here that oxygen from the air in the lungs passes through the alveoli walls into the blood. At the same time carbon dioxide, the waste product of the oxidation of glucose in the body cells, passes from the blood stream into the air sacs and is breathed out. This exchange of gases in the lungs is called *external respiration*. Thus the air breathed out contains more carbon dioxide and less oxygen than the air breathed in (see Table 3.3).

Table 3.3 The composition of air

Chemical composition of air	Approximate percentage in air breathed in	Approximate percentage in air breathed out
Nitrogen	78	78
Oxygen	20	17
Carbon dioxide	0·03	4
Inert gases	1	1
Water vapour	varies	increased

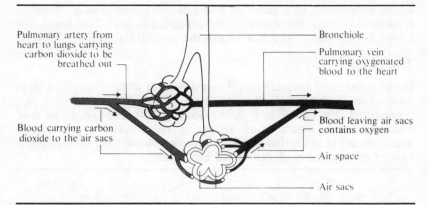

Fig. 3.7 The air sacs of the lungs showing the capillary network

Experiment 3.1 To show that more carbon dioxide is breathed out than is breathed in.

Using the apparatus shown in Fig. 3.8, breathe gently in and out through the T-piece at A. Air is forced in through the flask B and breathed out through flask C. Each flask contains an equal volume of lime water. Carbon dioxide turns lime water milky. The lime water in flask C becomes milky first, showing that there is more carbon dioxide in the air breathed out.

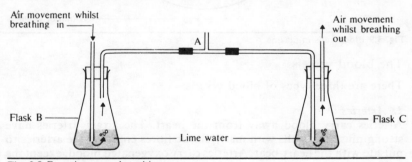

Fig. 3.8 Experiment on breathing

Experiment 3.2 The examination of the lungs and wind pipe of a sheep. From a butcher obtain a sheep's lungs with the wind pipe intact. Note the incomplete rings of cartilage in the trachea and bronchi, which hold the wind pipe open. Cut along one bronchus and follow its divisions into the lung tissue.

The circulatory system

Digested food and oxygen are both carried to the body cells in blood which is enclosed in a series of tubes called *blood vessels*. Blood is circulated through the vessels by the pumping action of the *heart*. The blood, blood vessels and heart form the circulatory system.

The blood

Blood consists of a watery liquid called *plasma* which contains a large number of *red blood cells*, a smaller number of *white cells* and fragmented cells known as *platelets* (see Fig. 3.9). The various parts of blood and their functions are shown in Table 3.4. The products of digestion are thus carried in solution in the blood plasma. Oxygen is carried as oxy-haemoglobin in red blood cells.

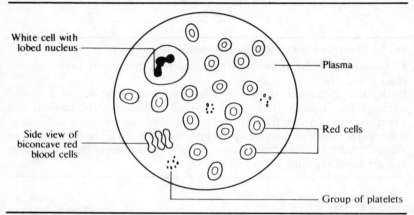

Fig. 3.9 Blood cells in plasma

The blood vessels

There are three types of blood vessels:

1. Arteries
Arteries carry blood away from the heart. The larger arteries have strong muscular walls with many elastic fibres enabling the arteries to pulsate with the heart-beat. Arteries carry oxygenated blood, except the pulmonary arteries which take de-oxygenated blood from the heart to the lungs.

2. Veins
Veins carry blood to the heart. They contain de-oxygenated blood, except the pulmonary veins which carry oxygenated blood from the lungs to the heart. The long veins, such as those in the limbs which carry blood upwards to the heart, have pocket-like valves on their inside walls to prevent blood from flowing backwards. If the vein becomes distended, the valves do not work and the condition is known as varicose veins.

3. Capillaries

Capillaries are very fine blood vessels which form a network between small arteries and small veins. Their walls are only one cell thick, and allow the passage of liquids and the diffusion of gases to and from the tissues. White blood cells squeeze their way between the cells of the capillary walls to fight infection in the tissues.

Table 3.4. Structure and functions of blood.

Part of blood	Description	Function
1. Plasma (the liquid part of blood)	A thin, yellowish, watery liquid	Transports dissolved substances including digested food, hormones and waste products such as carbon dioxide and urea. (Urea is formed in the liver from unwanted amino acids, and is later excreted in the urine by the kidneys.) Also carries red and white blood cells, and blood platelets
2. Red cells	Small biconcave cells with no nuclei. Live only 3 to 4 months. Are made in bone marrow. Contain haemoglobin, a compound of protein and iron, which makes the cells red	To carry oxygen from the lungs to the tissues. Oxygen combines with the haemoglobin to form oxy-haemoglobin which easily gives up oxygen in the tissues
3. White cells	Larger than red cells but fewer in number (500 red to 1 white)	To fight infection. The cells pass through the walls of blood capillaries to reach germs in the tissues. They surround bacteria and digest them
4. Platelets	Fragments of cells with no nuclei	To help in the clotting of blood

The heart

The heart is a hollow muscular organ which acts as a pump circulating blood through the blood vessels by contraction of the heart muscles. The contraction or heart-beat takes place about seventy to eighty times a minute but the rate is increased by exercise and by excitement. The heart is divided vertically into two distinct parts by a *septum* so that there is no connection between the left and right sides and each half acts as a separate pump (see Fig. 3.10).

The right side contains only de-oxygenated blood and the left side only oxygenated blood. Each side is divided into two cavities, thin-walled upper cavities called *atria* (or auricles) and thick-walled lower cavities called *ventricles*. Each atrium opens into the ventricle below it, the opening containing a valve which allows blood to flow in one direction only, from the atrium to the ventricle. The two atria contract together forcing blood into the ventricles. Contraction of the ventricles then forces blood into the large arteries through which it leaves the heart. Pocket-like semi-lunar valves in the inner walls of the arteries prevent the flow of blood back into the heart.

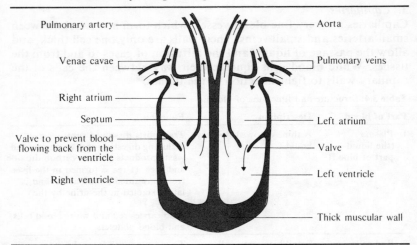

Fig. 3.10 The structure of the heart

The circulation of blood

De-oxygenated blood from all parts of the body flows through the veins into the right atrium. This blood contains carbon dioxide, and also digested food which has entered the blood from the small intestine (see Fig. 3.11). Contraction of the right atrium forces the blood through the valve into the right ventricle, which in turn contracts, driving the blood through the pulmonary artery to the lungs. Here carbon dioxide leaves the blood and oxygen enters. The oxygenated blood still containing digested food returns to the left atrium along the pulmonary veins. Contraction of the atrium forces blood into the left ventricle. From here it is pumped into the main artery, the aorta, which has branches to all parts of the body including the skin and hair follicles. In the capillary networks of the body tissues oxygen and food are transferred to the cells, and waste carbon dioxide enters the blood to be returned to the heart.

The circulation of the blood is shown in Fig. 3.11. There is a double circulation.

1. **The pulmonary circulation** from the right ventricle to the lungs and back to the left atrium.

   Heart ⟶ lungs ⟶ heart.

2. **The systemic circulation** from the left ventricle to the body tissues back to the right atrium.

   Heart ⟶ body tissues ⟶ heart.

The blood supply to the head

Soon after leaving the heart, the aorta branches to supply the arms and the head. The two *common carotid arteries*, which supply the head, run

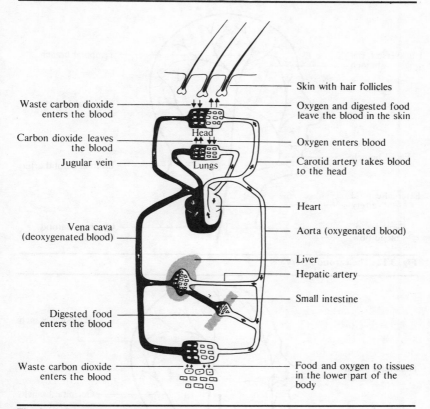

Waste carbon dioxide enters the blood

Carbon dioxide leaves the blood

Jugular vein

Head

Lungs

Vena cava (deoxygenated blood)

Digested food enters the blood

Waste carbon dioxide enters the blood

Skin with hair follicles

Oxygen and digested food leave the blood in the skin

Oxygen enters blood

Carotid artery takes blood to the head

Heart

Aorta (oxygenated blood)

Liver

Hepatic artery

Small intestine

Food and oxygen to tissues in the lower part of the body

Fig. 3.11 The circulation of the blood

up through the neck, one along each side of the wind-pipe. At about the level of the Adam's apple they each divide into an internal and an external branch. The *internal carotid arteries* pass through openings in the temporal bones of the skull, to take blood to the brain. The *external carotid arteries* remain outside the skull and continue one along each side of the head, branching to supply the muscles and skin of the face and scalp. The branches of the external carotid artery are shown in Fig. 3.12. The temporal branch takes blood to the scalp. It divides into capillaries in the skin of the scalp and supplies blood to the hair follicles. These capillaries join to form the temporal branch of the *jugular vein* which takes de-oxygenated blood from the head to the heart as shown in Fig. 3.13.

The blood supply to a hair papilla

As blood passes through the capillary network in the hair papilla, a liquid oozes out through the porous walls of the capillaries to bathe the

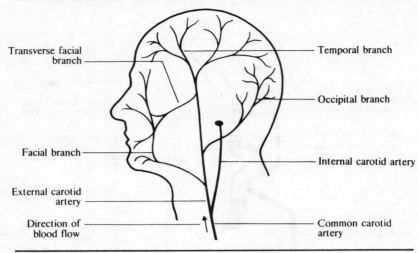

Transverse facial branch

Temporal branch

Occipital branch

Facial branch

Internal carotid artery

External carotid artery

Direction of blood flow

Common carotid artery

Fig. 3.12 The carotid artery

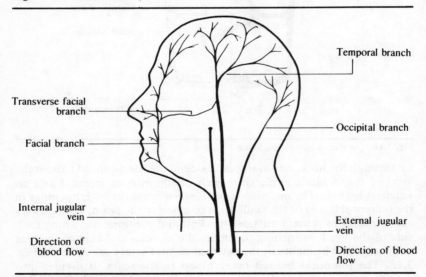

Temporal branch

Transverse facial branch

Facial branch

Occipital branch

Internal jugular vein

External jugular vein

Direction of blood flow

Direction of blood flow

Fig. 3.13 The jugular vein

surrounding cells. The liquid is *tissue fluid* and is similar to blood plasma. Oxygen which is released from the haemoglobin of red blood cells and the products of digestion (amino acids, fatty acids and glucose) are carried by tissue fluid to the cells round the hair papilla, so enabling growth of new hair to take place (see Fig. 3.14). Some of the tissue fluid re-enters the capillaries carrying waste carbon dioxide and some flows away into other channels called *lymph vessels*. This exchange of gases in the tissues is known as *tissue respiration* or *internal respiration*.

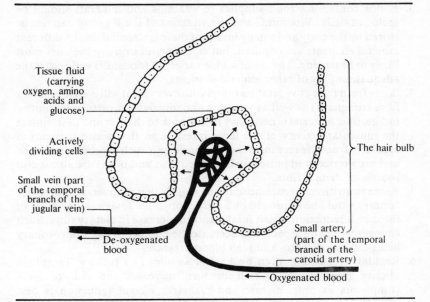

Fig. 3.14 The blood supply to a hair papilla

The growing hair receives nourishment only through the blood stream. Substances applied externally to the hair shaft do not supply nourishment as the hair cells are then dead and fully keratinised. These substances may, of course, improve the condition of the hair. The nutrition of hair thus depends on diet and the circulation of blood to the scalp. The circulation may be improved by massage. This is often carried out in a salon using hand massage or by use of a vibro-massage machine.

Diet

A satisfactory daily diet may be obtained by considering the following points:
1. The diet should include as wide a variety of foods as possible.
2. The protein content of a meal should be considered first. Small helpings of protein included in every meal are better than one large helping of protein food per day. Proteins are used most economically in the body if animal and vegetable protein foods are eaten together at the same meal rather than on separate occasions, and if foods containing some carbohydrate are consumed along with the protein. It must be emphasised that although protein is required for building hair, increasing the amount of protein in the diet does not necessarily increase hair growth. The extra protein may be used in other parts of the body or be broken down to provide energy.

3. Foods containing good supplies of vitamins and minerals should be included daily. Vitamin C and the vitamins of the B group can not be stored by the body and a daily intake of these is essential. Many different mineral elements are required, but calcium and iron are the ones most likely to be lacking. The use of a wide variety of foodstuffs will ensure the adequate supply of other mineral elements.

4. Some fresh fruit or vegetables taken with every meal will provide dietary fibre (roughage) as well as vitamins and minerals. A certain amount of indigestible material is necessary to add bulk to the diet and to stimulate the muscular activity of the large intestine so that waste is removed regularly from the rectum. Whole grain cereals such as wholemeal flour and brown rice, and pulses such as dried peas and beans are also useful sources of dietary fibre.

5. Recent nutritional recommendations suggest that the average diet of this country would be improved by a reduction in the total amount of fat in the diet, a reduction of salt intake and an increase in dietary fibre. Such changes would be expected to decrease the number of cases of coronary heart disease, diabetes and high blood pressure.

6. Regular over-eating, even by a small amount at a time, will result in obesity (over-weight) which in turn increases the risk of such complaints as heart disease and diabetes. Weight reduction is best carried out by a slight reduction of food intake by eating smaller helpings, always taking care to maintain essential nutrients especially protein, calcium and iron. The use of crash diets or unbalanced 'slimming diets' which can only be maintained for short periods of time should be avoided. Any weight lost by following such diets may be quickly regained if the consumption of food is later returned to its former intake. Additional exercise may assist weight reduction and improve general health.

Questions

1. By what pathway does oxygen from the air reach the capillaries in the hair papillae? Why is a supply of oxygen required in the papillae?
2. By what pathway does protein food such as egg reach the capillaries of the hair papilla in the form of amino acids? Why are amino acids required in the hair papillae?
3. Explain how lack of iron in the diet may lead to anaemia. Why does anaemia cause a feeling of tiredness?
4. Suggest foods for a day's menu including a packed lunch. List the nutrients provided by each food.
5. What is meant by:
   (a) digestion;   (b) tissue fluid;   (c) a catalyst;   (d) internal and external respiration;   (e) oxidation?

Chapter 4

The shape and structure
of the head

The shape of the face and head, and the shape and proportions of the main features of the face are important factors to be considered when choosing a suitable hairstyle for a particular client. These shapes are largely determined by:
1. The bone structure of the skull (see Fig. 4.1 and Fig. 4.2).
2. The muscles covering the bones of the face (see Fig. 4.3 and Fig. 4.4).

The skull

The skull consists of two parts: (1) the *cranium*, which is a protective box holding the brain, and (2) the *face*. There are eight bones in the cranium and fourteen in the face. The only movable bone in the skull is the lower jaw which is hinged to allow chewing and talking. All the other bones are held rigidly together by saw-edged joints or *sutures*.

The bones of the cranium

The bones of the cranium are as follows:
1. **The frontal bone** forms the forehead and the front part of the top of the skull.
2. **A pair of parietal bones** join down the mid-line of the top of the skull.
3. **The occipital bone** forms the back and part of the base of the skull. In it is a large opening, the foramen magnum, through which passes the spinal cord.
4. **A pair of temporal bones** form the lower part of the side of the cranium and contain cavities for the ear passages. A portion of the temporal bone juts out to join the cheek bone forming the *zygomatic arch* which may be felt just in front of the lower part of the ear. The mastoid process is a projection from the temporal bone forming a small lump just behind the ear. This surrounds and protects the inner part of the ear and also forms a point of attachment for the sterno-mastoid muscle in the neck.
5. **The sphenoid bone** occupies most of the base of the cranium. It is shaped like a bat with its extended wing tips forming part of each side of the skull between the temporal and frontal bones.

6. **The ethmoid bone**, a small irregularly shaped bone, forms part of the base of the cranium, the roof of the nose and the inner wall of the *orbits* (eye-sockets). This bone is not shown in the diagrams.

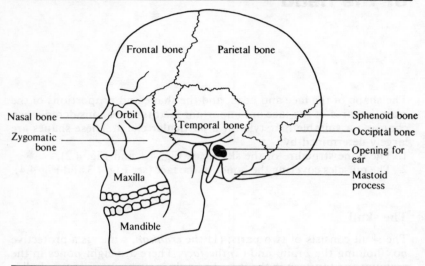

Fig. 4.1 Side view of the skull

The bones of the face

The following bones give shape to the face:

1. **A pair of small nasal bones** make the bridge of the nose. The rest of the nose contains cartilage which is softer and more flexible than bone. This cartilage determines the shape of the tip of the nose.
2. **A pair of zygomatic bones** (malar) form the cheek bones which may be felt just below the eyes. The zygomatic arches join the cheek bones and the temporal bones providing a place of attachment for the muscles raising the upper lip.
3. **The two superior maxillary bones** or maxillae form the upper jaw and hold the upper teeth.
4. **The inferior maxillary bone** or mandible forms the lower jaw and holds the lower teeth.

The other seven bones of the face are inside the skull behind the nose, in the roof of the mouth, and inside the orbits and have no influence on the shape of the face.

The muscles of the head and neck

The bones of the face are covered by layers of muscle or flesh which together with the skin and its underlying layer of fatty tissue give roundness to the contours of the face. Lack of subcutaneous fat may

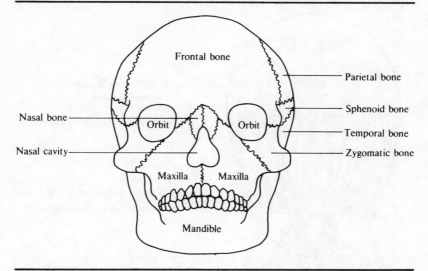

Fig. 4.2 Front view of the skull

make the cheeks look hollow. The contours of the face change with age due to sagging muscles and decreased elasticity of the skin causing wrinkles to appear.

Muscles work by contracting in length. They can pull but never push. Muscles may be attached:

(a) to bone at both ends, e.g. the muscles of the limbs;
(b) to bône at one end and skin at the other, e.g. the muscles raising the upper lip extend from the lip to the zygomatic arch;
(c) to the skin at both ends, e.g. the muscles of expression in the face.

The muscles of facial expression

Circular muscles (the orbicularis oculi) surround each eye enabling it to be screwed up or opened wide. A similar circular muscle (the orbicularis oris) surrounds the mouth for movement of the lips in speaking, pouting, whistling, etc. Groups of small muscles radiate from this circular muscle to raise and lower the angle of the mouth when smiling or looking 'down in the mouth'. Small muscles just above the eyes cause frowning and other muscles wrinkle the nose.

The muscles of mastication

The masseter and the temporalis muscles enable chewing and biting to take place. The temporalis lies over the temporal bone and joins the jaw after passing in front of the ear. The masseter joins the jaw to the zygomatic arch.

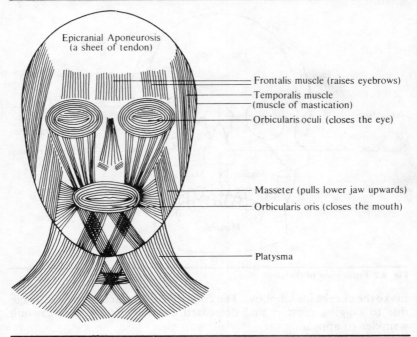

Epicranial Aponeurosis
(a sheet of tendon)

Frontalis muscle (raises eyebrows)

Temporalis muscle
(muscle of mastication)

Orbicularis oculi (closes the eye)

Masseter (pulls lower jaw upwards)

Orbicularis oris (closes the mouth)

Platysma

Fig. 4.3 The muscles of the face

The muscles of the neck

There are three main muscles in the neck:
1. The sterno-mastoid is used in turning the head.
2. The trapezius raises the shoulders.
3. The platysma is a thin sheet of muscle just under the skin of the neck. It stretches from the mouth, under the chin and down the neck to the chest. It is used in swallowing and also in the expression of sudden fear.

The shape of the head and neck

The variation of head shape in different people is due largely to differences in the shape of the bones of the skull. The layer of soft tissue covering the skull is relatively thin and has little effect on head shape except in the more muscular areas of the cheeks and chin. Good hair styling depends on a preliminary study of the shape of the client's head and neck. The choice of style should enhance the appearance of the client by highlighting the pleasing points of head structure, and to some extent decreasing the prominence of any undesirable features. To achieve this

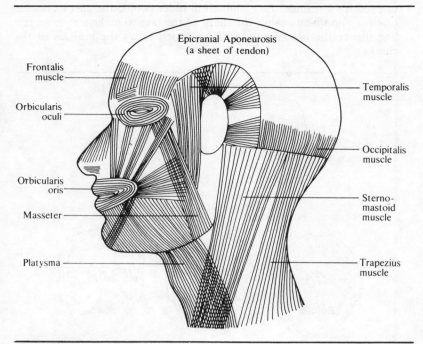

Fig. 4.4 The muscles of the head and neck

the hairdresser must study the shape of the head and neck both from the front and in profile. The shapes are perhaps best seen when the hair is wet and lies close to the head.

Viewing from the front the following features should be noted.

1. *The shape of the face* (see Fig. 4.5). The face is the lower front portion of the head, bounded above by the hair line on the forehead and outlined by the cheeks and chin. Basic face shapes are usually regarded as round, oval, square, oblong, diamond-shaped, heart-shaped and triangular though many faces are a mixture of shapes. Face shape depends largely on the length of the face from the hairline to the chin, the width of the face between the zygomatic arches and at forehead level, the shape of the mandible (lower jaw), and the amount of muscle (flesh) in the cheeks.

   The widest part of the face is usually determined by the zygomatic arches which join the zygomatic bones to the temporal bones on each side of the head. They are particularly prominent in diamond- and heart-shaped faces. The length and width of the face are approximately equal in square and round faces, whilst the length is greater than the width in oval and oblong ones. Square jaws are typical of square and oblong faces, whereas pointed jaws occur in diamond, heart-shaped and triangular faces. The presence of well-formed cheek muscles tends to produce a rounder face, though in older people the cheek muscles often sag and may change the shape of the face to make a squarer jaw line (hence the need for face lifting which raises the muscles of the cheeks).

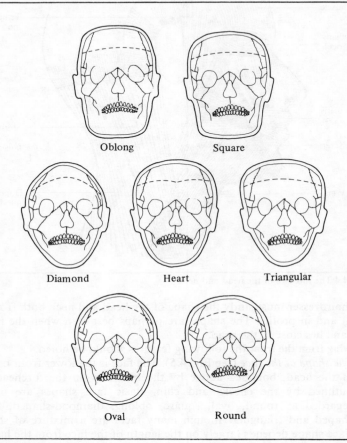

Fig. 4.5 Face shapes

2. *The dome of the skull.* The upper part of the skull may have a high dome or may be quite flattened. The height of the head above the forehead hair line must be taken into consideration before styling.
3. *The prominence and size of the ears.*
4. *The length and width of the neck.* The sterno-mastoid and trapezius muscles contribute to the width of the neck, the platysma at the front of the neck usually consisting only of a very thin sheet of muscle. Neck lengths vary considerably although the basic bone structure always consists of seven vertebrae.

In profile (see Fig. 4.6) the following features should be observed.
1. *The prominence of the nose.*
2. *The shape of the chin.* The chin may recede or be prominent depending on the shape of the mandible and the amount of muscle at the tip of the chin. In old age, loss of teeth and the contraction of the mouth tissues may contribute to the prominence of the chin.
3. *The prominence of the frontal bone in the forehead.*
4. *The shape of the back of the skull.* The size of the hollow at the nape depends on the shape of the occipital bone at the back of the skull and the angle at which the neck vertebrae meet the base of the skull.

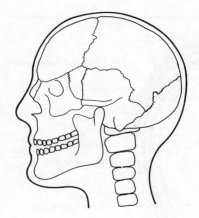 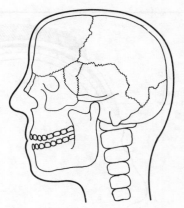

(a) High dome
    Occipital area rounded
    Hollow nape
    Receding forehead
    Prominent chin
    Small nose

(b) Dome of skull flattened
    Occipital area flattened
    No hollow at nape
    Prominent forehead
    Receding chin
    Prominent nose.

Fig. 4.6 Features of heads in profile

The scalp

The top of the head has no muscular covering. Lying between the skin and the skull is a broad strong sheet of non-elastic fibrous tissue or tendon called the epicranial aponeurosis (see Fig. 4.7).

The scalp consists of all the tissues covering the top of the cranium, that is:

1. The skin with the scalp hair.
2. The connective tissue which firmly attaches the skin to the epicranial aponeurosis.
3. The epicranial aponeurosis itself.
4. The very loose connective tissue between the epicranial aponeurosis and the bone of the skull.

The epicranial aponeurosis is held by the frontalis muscle at the front of the head and the occipitalis muscle at the back. At the sides it is attached to the temporalis muscles. It is also held very loosely, by connective tissue, to the bone of the skull so that the whole scalp can be moved over the surface of the skull. This movement may be noticed during shampooing. Some people are able to move the epicranial aponeurosis at will by alternately contracting the frontalis and the occipitalis muscles.

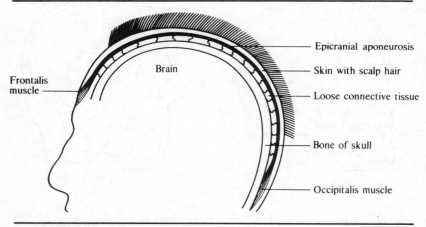

Fig. 4.7 The structure of the scalp

Questions

1. Draw a diagram of the skull as seen from above.
2. By considering the structure of the scalp explain what is meant by a 'tight scalp' and a 'loose scalp'.
3. What is the function of:
   (a) the skull;   (b) the zygomatic arches;   (c) the orbicularis oris;   (d) the mastoid process.
4. Explain what is meant by:
   (a) the spinal cord;   (b) the orbits;   (c) cartilage;
   (d) the epicranial aponeurosis.
5. Explain:
   (a) what causes the skin to wrinkle;
   (b) how some people are able to move their own scalp;
   (c) why the contours of the face change with age.

Part 2
The salon

Chapter 5

Mirrors in the salon

Mirrors have many uses in a salon other than providing the hairdresser with a view of the client, or giving the client a back view of the final result of the hairdresser's art. They can add light to a salon, alter its apparent shape or size, give decorative effects and even enable the hairdresser to see round corners. Careful placing of mirrors is essential, if such benefits are to be obtained and unpleasant effects caused by bad siting are to be avoided.

The placing of mirrors depends on the properties of light. We can only see an object when light passes from that object to our eyes. The light takes the shortest route, that is, it travels in a straight line between the object and the eye. This law – *light travels in straight lines* – is the basis of the study of mirrors and of the diagrams drawn to indicate the pathway of rays or beams of light.

Light may change direction

If a beam of light which has been travelling through air meets a different substance such as polished metal, glass or water its direction is usually changed at the surface. The beam may be either *reflected* or *refracted*.

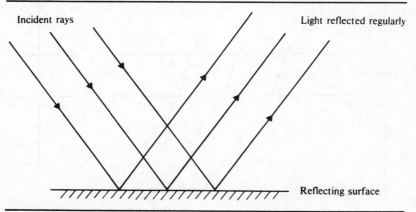

Incident rays   Light reflected regularly

Reflecting surface

Fig. 5.1 Uniform reflection

Reflection

At a smooth surface the light may be reflected regularly (see Fig. 5.1). A surface from which a high proportion of light is reflected regularly is glossy or has lustre. At a rough surface the light may be reflected in

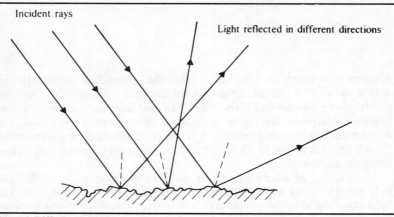

Incident rays

Light reflected in different directions

Fig. 5.2 Diffusion by reflection

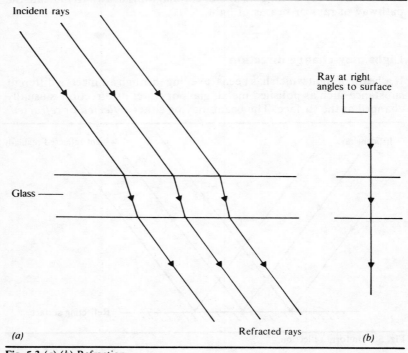

Incident rays

Ray at right angles to surface

Glass ———

(a)

Refracted rays

(b)

Fig. 5.3 (*a*) (*b*) Refraction

many different directions. The light is scattered or *diffused*. A surface from which light is reflected diffusely appears matt or dull. The rougher the surface of a hair the duller it appears (see Fig. 5.2).

Refraction

If a substance is transparent, like a sheet of glass, light passing through it is bent or refracted (see Fig. 5.3*a*). The light changes direction on entering the glass and again on leaving, unless the rays are at right angles to the glass when the beam goes straight through (see Fig. 5.3*b*). If the surface of the glass is rough, the light is diffused as well as being refracted. If the diffusion is great enough, the glass becomes translucent and objects cannot be seen clearly through the glass although light is passing through it (see Fig. 5.4).

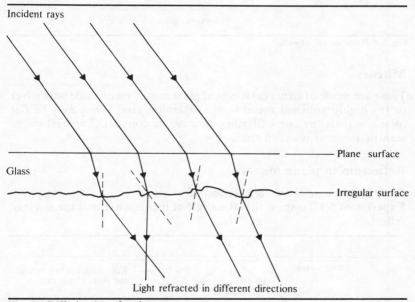

Fig. 5.4 Diffusion by refraction

How we see objects

We see objects when light is reflected from the surface of the object to our eyes (see Fig. 5.5). The light from the object passes through the lens of the eye and is focused on the retina at the back of the eye where an image is formed. The endings of the optic nerve in the retina are thus stimulated. Impulses pass along the nerve to the brain, causing sight. The use of both eyes together gives two slightly different views of an object, so producing a three-dimensional impression which gives depth to our vision.

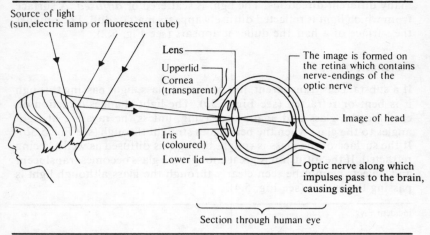

Source of light
(sun, electric lamp or fluorescent tube)

Lens

Upperlid

Cornea
(transparent)

Iris
(coloured)

Lower lid

The image is formed on
the retina which contains
nerve-endings of the
optic nerve

Image of head

Optic nerve along which
impulses pass to the brain,
causing sight

Section through human eye

Fig. 5.5 How we see objects

Mirrors

These are made of either (a) sheets of glass coated on one side with silver
or (b) highly polished metal such as stainless steel. They may be flat
(plane mirrors) or curved (either concave or convex). The 'reflection'
seen in a mirror is called the *image*.

Reflection in plane mirrors

1. At what angle is the light reflected?
Experiment 5.1 To show that the angle of incidence equals the angle of
reflection.

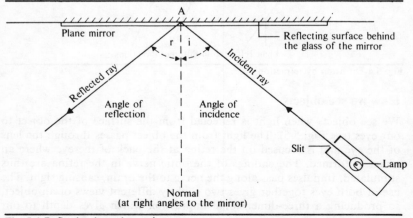

A

Plane mirror

r   i

Reflecting surface behind
the glass of the mirror

Reflected ray

Incident ray

Angle of
reflection

Angle of
incidence

Slit

Lamp

Normal
(at right angles to the mirror)

Fig. 5.6 Reflection in a plane mirror

Support a plane mirror vertically on a sheet of paper on a line marking the position of the reflecting surface (see Fig. 5.6). Using a ray box, arrange a narrow beam of light to strike the mirror at A. Mark the positions of the incident ray and reflected ray by putting pencil marks in the middle of the beam at several points along its length. Remove all the apparatus, and draw the normal at A at right angles to the mirror and rule lines along the two rays. Measure the angle of incidence and the angle of reflection. Repeat several times using different angles of incidence. It will be found that in each case *the angle of incidence equals the angle of reflection*. So the reflected ray leaves the mirror at the same angle as that at which the incident ray meets the mirror.

2. *Where is the image?*

The position of the image in the mirror can be found by the following construction (see Fig. 5.7). The line RS represents a plane mirror and O an object in front. The two lines OM and ON are drawn at different angles to the mirror to represent rays of light travelling from the object to the mirror. By drawing the normals at M and N, measuring the angles of incidence and making the angles of reflection equal to the angles of incidence in each case, the reflected rays ML and NP are obtained. The lines LM and PN extended behind the mirror meet at I. An eye at L would see the image of O in the direction LM, and similarly looking from P the image of O would be seen in the direction PN. If it may be seen in both these directions, the image must be at I.

So the image of object O is at I.

By joining IO it is found that IT = TO

Thus the image in a plane mirror is as far behind the mirror as the object is in front.

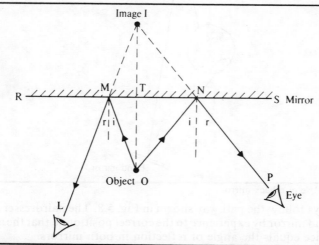

Fig. 5.7 Position of an image in a plane mirror

3. How big is the image?

By observation it can be seen that in *a plane mirror the image is always the same size as the object.*

4. Left-handed or right-handed?

Your client may startle you by saying 'Oh, are you left-handed?' when you are busy cutting with scissors in your right hand. Or if you have a new ring on your right hand she may ask 'Have you become engaged?'. She does this when looking through the mirror on the dressing table in front of her. A mirror appears to turn an object round so that the right side of the object appears as the left side of the image. This is known as *lateral inversion.*

Experiment 5.2. To show lateral inversion
(a) Hold your left ear with your left hand and notice that in the mirror your image appears to be holding your right ear with your right hand.
(b) Write your name on a paper whilst looking at the paper through a mirror.
(c) Write your name on a paper using wet ink. Blot it and look at the blotting paper. Hold the blotting paper up to a mirror to read it.

Using plane mirrors in a salon

To enable the client to see the back of her head

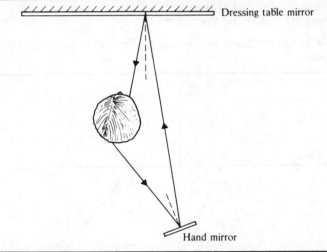

Fig. 5.8 Use of a back mirror

The rays follow the pathway shown in Fig. 5.8. The hairdresser adjusts the hand mirror by experience to the correct position so that the angle of incidence equals the angle of reflection in both mirrors.

To make the salon appear larger

Since the image is as far behind the mirror as the object is in front, a large mirror covering one wall of a salon would make the salon appear twice as big (see Fig. 5.9).

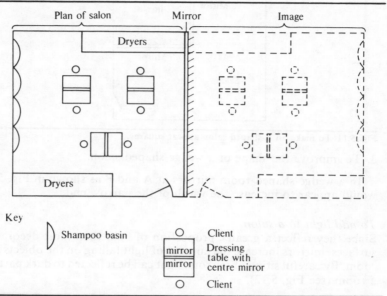

Key

) Shampoo basin   O   Client

[mirror / mirror] Dressing table with centre mirror

O   Client

Fig. 5.9 A wall-mirror increases the apparent size of the salon

To make a salon appear different in shape

1. A long narrow salon can be made to appear twice as wide (see Fig. 5.10).

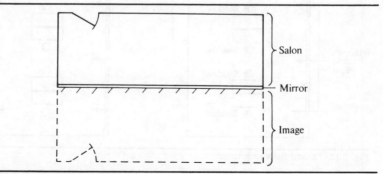

Fig. 5.10 To make a long, narrow salon appear wider

2. An L-shaped salon may be made to look square (see Fig. 5.11).

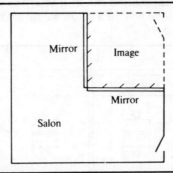

Fig. 5.11 To make an L-shaped salon appear square

3. To improve the shape of a wedge-shaped salon.

In a wedge-shaped room mirrors at A and B as shown in Fig. 5.13 would appear to increase the width of the narrow end.

To add light to a salon
Since they reflect a greater proportion of light than most decorative surfaces, mirrors increase the amount of light falling on the objects in a room. By careful siting of mirrors, light can be reflected to dark parts of a room (see Fig. 5.12).

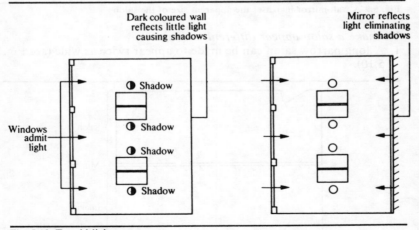

Fig. 5.12 To add light to a room

To enable a hairdresser to see round a corner
A salon may be shaped so that the door through which the clients enter cannot be seen from all parts of the room. By careful siting of mirrors, the hairdresser may avoid having to leave a client to see who has entered

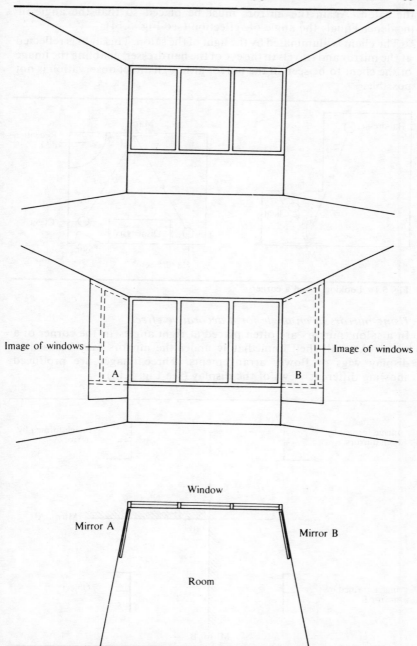

Fig. 5.13 To make a room appear wider

the salon. Again the mirrors must be placed so that the angle of incidence equals the angle of reflection (see Fig. 5.14).

The client is illuminated by the light of the salon. This light is reflected at the mirror and travels to the eye of the hairdresser, enabling the image of the client to be seen in the mirror although direct observation is not possible.

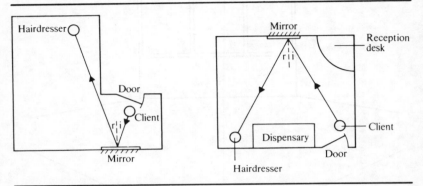

Fig. 5.14 Looking round a corner

Using mirrors at an angle for a decorative effect

In a salon, mirrors are often placed at right angles in the corner of a room. A small shelf immediately under the mirrors may be used to display wigs or flower arrangements. Three images are produced showing different views of the display (see Fig. 5.15).

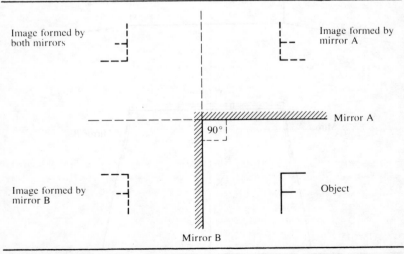

Fig. 5.15 Multiple images

Experiment 5.3 To find the number of images produced by inclined mirrors

Arrange two mirrors vertically at an angle. Place an object in front of the mirrors and count the number of images produced at various angles. It will be found that the smaller the angle between the mirrors the greater the number of images (see Table 5.1).

Table 5.1 Images produced by mirrors at an angle.

Angle between mirrors (in degrees)	Number of images
180	1
120	2
90	3
72	4
60	5
40	8
30	11

The use of curved mirrors

1. Concave mirrors

These mirrors reflect light from the inside of the curve. They are used as make-up or shaving mirrors to give a magnified image when used near to the face (see Fig. 5.16).

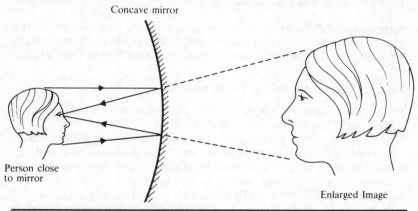

Concave mirror

Person close to mirror

Enlarged Image

Fig. 5.16 Reflection by a concave mirror

Experiment 5.4 To examine the image produced by a concave mirror

Hold a small concave mirror at arm's length and look for your own image. Move the mirror by tilting it or by bending your arm slightly until you see a clear image of your eye. The image will probably be inverted (if it is not, choose another mirror with a greater curvature). Gradually bring the mirror towards your face. The image becomes blurred until the mirror is near to the face, when a clear, erect and much enlarged image will be produced.

2. Convex mirrors.

These mirrors reflect light from the outside of the curve. This type of mirror may be used to give a wide field of view of the whole salon from a single point, for supervisory purposes. Convex mirrors are often used in powder compacts to give a small view of the whole face (see Fig. 5.17).

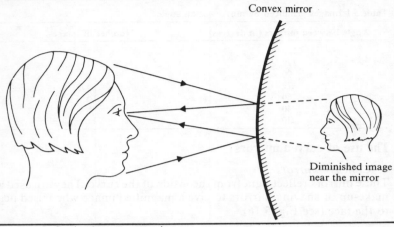

Fig. 5.17 Reflection by a convex mirror

Experiment 5.5 To examine the image produced in a convex mirror
Hold a small convex mirror at arm's length and gradually bring it nearer to your face. The image is always erect and smaller than the object.

General comments on the use of mirrors

1. Too many mirrors in a small salon may present a confusing picture and make the salon look crowded.
2. Parallel mirrors produce a large number of repeating images extending back a considerable way behind the mirror and this may be disturbing to some people. Mirrors opposite to each other on the salon walls should thus be avoided.
3. Mirrors should be carefully sited with respect to lighting fixtures to avoid glare. If bright lights are visible in mirrors they could be irritating to the eyes. Lights over mirrors should shine on the client not on the mirror itself and be well shaded from the client's eyes.
4. Mirrors extending to the floor are often dangerous as people tend to walk into them.
5. Mirrors over shampoo basins are subject to condensation. Mirror lights slightly heat the glass and therefore help to prevent the deposit of moisture.
6. Mirrors should be kept clean and free from finger marks and smears. Remember that each mark is seen twice, once as an image. Mirrors may be cleaned with methylated spirit, and this is particularly useful for the removal of spots of lacquer.

Questions

1. Draw the mirror images corresponding to the objects shown in Fig. 5.18.

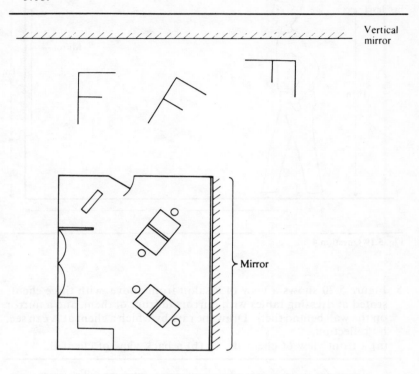

Fig. 5.18 Question 1

2. Draw a plan of your salon showing the position of all wall mirrors. Explain the purpose of the mirrors. In your opinion are they being used to the best advantage? If not, suggest where they could be resited or where others could be added.

3. Describe the type of image which would be produced by using (a) a plane, (b) a convex and (c) a concave mirror in a powder compact. Which type do you consider to be most satisfactory? Give the reason for your choice.

4. A mirror is placed vertically on a wall at the height shown in Fig. 5.19. Draw a diagram showing the position of the image of the person at A. By drawing in the rays, show how it is possible for him to see his own feet.

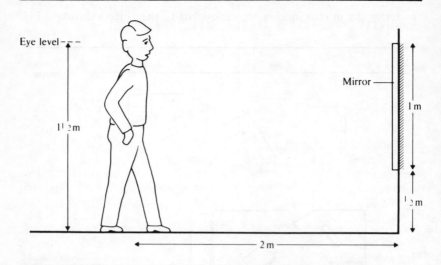

Eye level

$1\frac{1}{2}$ m

Mirror

1 m

$\frac{1}{2}$ m

2 m

Fig. 5.19 Question 4

5. Figure 5.20 shows a view of a salon from above, with three clients seated at dressing tables with mirrors in front of them, and a mirror on the wall behind them. Draw the rays by which a client at A can see, by reflection,
   (a) a front view of client B;   (b) a back view of client B.

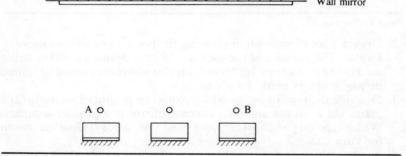

Wall mirror

A ○   ○   ○ B

Fig. 5.20 Question 5

Chapter 6

Comfortable air conditions in the salon

The human body has an automatic mechanism to keep it at constant temperature. Changes in the temperature and humidity of the surrounding air may upset this mechanism, causing discomfort due to overheating or excessive cooling. Discomfort may also result from the presence of fumes such as ammonia or lacquer fumes in the air, and these may irritate the lining of the air passages. If the air in a busy salon is not changed frequently, excessive humidity and changes in the composition of the atmosphere lead to 'stuffiness', and the occupants feel tired or faint. These factors affecting the comfort of the people in a salon can largely be controlled by heating and ventilation systems, though clothing, too, plays a part in the control of body heat. To understand these topics, a knowledge of the nature and effects of heat is required.

What is heat?

The molecules of a substance are in constant motion and therefore possess mechanical energy. Heat, too, is a form of energy and if a substance is heated energy passes from the source of heat to the substance, making its molecules move faster. Thus heat energy is converted to mechanical energy. The speed of the molecules increases as the temperature rises.

The effect of heat

If a substance is heated, one or more of the following changes may take place:

1. Heating may cause a change of state
Substances may exist in three different states as solids, liquids or gases. Heating often causes a substance to change from one of these states to another.

A solid has a definite shape, for its molecules are held closely together by strong forces of attraction. Although the molecules remain approximately in the same position within the solid, they are in constant vibration. When a solid is heated, the molecules vibrate more quickly until they finally break away from one another and the solid *melts*, changing its state to become a liquid.

The molecules in a *liquid* move about more freely than those in a solid. They constantly bounce back from the sides of the vessel containing them and also frequently bump into each other. When a liquid is heated, some of the molecules may gain sufficient speed, at any temperature, to escape from the liquid when they strike its surface. The liquid thus changes to a gaseous state, and *evaporation* has taken place. This process takes place most rapidly when the temperature reaches boiling point.

The molecules in *a gas* have more energy than those in a liquid and so move about more rapidly. A gas occupies all the space available to it.

Similarly loss of heat may cause change of state from a gas to a liquid (*condensation*) and from a liquid to a solid (*solidification*). Changes of state are physical changes. No new substances are formed, the same substance merely changing its form.

Changes of state may be summarised as shown in Fig. 6.1.

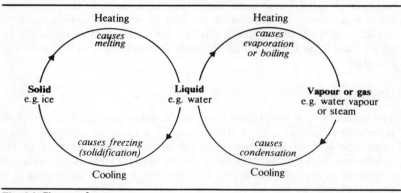

Fig. 6.1 Change of state

2. Heating causes substances to expand

In general, solids, liquids and gases will all expand during heating and contract again during cooling. Water cooled between $4°C$ and $0°C$ is an exception to the rule, as water cooled within this range of temperatures expands. It is this expansion which causes the bursting of pipes when the water in them freezes. Expansion and contraction are physical changes.

3. Heating may cause chemical changes to take place

Heat often starts or speeds up chemical changes. Some substances such as hydrogen peroxide are decomposed by heat.

Hydrogen peroxide $\xrightarrow{\text{heat}}$ water + oxygen

The steamer or accelerator is used in the salon to provide heat to speed the chemical reactions which take place in bleaching, perming and colouring hair.

4. Heat causes a rise in temperature

This rule applies except whilst substances are changing state. If a thermometer is placed in a beaker of cold water which is then heated until the water boils, the temperature will rise to 100°C but will then remain steady whilst the water turns to steam, although the water is still being heated. This heat, which causes change of state without raising the temperature, is called *latent heat*.

The measurement of temperature

The temperature or 'hotness' of a substance is usually measured by a liquid-in-glass *thermometer*, the working of which depends on the principle that liquids expand evenly on heating and contract quickly during cooling. The liquids used are usually mercury or coloured alcohol, which are enclosed in a glass bulb and on expanding move up a fine capillary tube running the length of the stem of the thermometer. The *Celsius* (Centigrade) scale is used for modern thermometers. The scale is divided into 100 divisions between the melting point of ice which is 0°C and the boiling point of water which is 100°C. Temperature is important because it determines the direction of flow of heat between two objects. Heat always flows from an object at a high temperature to one at a low temperature and never in the opposite direction.

A *clinical thermometer* is used to measure body temperature (see Fig 6.2). It should be held under the tongue for about one minute before being read. As cooling of the thermometer takes place, the mercury in the bulb contracts from a constriction in the capillary tube, leaving the mercury thread intact and enabling the reading to be made at leisure. The mercury thread should be rejoined before the thermometer is used again, by giving it a sharp jerk.

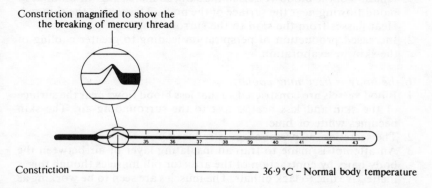

Constriction magnified to show the the breaking of mercury thread

Constriction

36·9°C – Normal body temperature

Fig. 6.2 A clinical thermometer

The regulation of body temperature

The body attempts to keep its own temperature constant at 36·9°C by equalising the heat gained and the heat lost by the body.

The body gains heat from:
1. The oxidation of food in the body tissues. Heat production by this method is increased with bodily activity or exercise.
2. External sources such as the sun or heating appliances.

The body loses heat by:
1. The passage of heat from the skin to the surrounding air since the body is usually at a higher temperature than the air.
2. Respiration, since the air breathed out is usually warmer than the air breathed in.
3. The cooling effect of evaporation of perspiration from the surface of the skin. Latent heat is taken from the skin to enable the change of state to take place.

Experiment 6.1 To show the cooling effect of evaporation
Support a 0°–100°C thermometer in a burette stand and note the room temperature. Surround the bulb of the thermometer with cotton wool and fasten it with thread or an elastic band. Dip the cotton wool into ether and note the lowering of the temperature as the ether evaporates. Ether is a volatile substance so evaporates quickly at room temperature. Latent heat is required to change the state of the ether from a liquid to a vapour. This heat is taken from the surroundings – in this case from the thermometer – and the reading is lowered.

The body reacts automatically to moderate change in the surrounding conditions.

If the body is becoming too hot:
It increases heat losses by:
1. Dilation of the blood vessels in the skin, so increasing the amount of blood flowing near the surface of the body. This makes the skin red. Heat passes from the skin to the surrounding air.
2. Increased production of perspiration leading to greater cooling of the skin by evaporation.

If the body is becoming cooler:
1. Blood vessels are constricted so that less blood flows near the surface of the skin and less heat is lost to the surrounding air. The skin becomes white or blue.
2. The secretion of perspiration is reduced.
3. An attempt is made to trap an insulating layer of air between the body hairs by contraction of the arrector pili muscles though this is ineffective due to lack of hair. The muscles are seen to be working as

contraction pulls the skin into goose pimples as well as raising the hairs.

4. Heat is produced by the muscular activity involved in shivering.

Air conditions affecting the comfort of people in a salon

There are four main factors affecting the comfort of the occupants of a room:

1. The air temperature

Room temperature should be kept constant at between 18°C and 21°C, by regulation of heating appliances and ventilation. If room temperature is too low clients will lose heat too quickly and feel cold. This will most probably occur early in the day if the salon has not been heated. The continual use of hair dryers and other heat-producing equipment tends to make the salon warmer as the day's work proceeds. As the room becomes warmer the rate of loss of heat from the surface of the skin decreases and the body may become uncomfortably warm. This factor is also affected by the type of clothing worn in the salon.

A wall thermometer is useful so that room temperature may be checked and heating and ventilation adjusted accordingly. The thermometer should be sited away from direct sunlight and other sources of heat such as radiators and hair dryers.

2. Humidity

If the humidity of the air is too low, the mucous membranes lining the nose and throat become uncomfortably dry and in this state are easily infected. In a salon, however, the humidity tends to be high due to:

(a) steam from the use of steamers and from hot water used for shampooing;

(b) evaporation of water during hair drying and the drying of towels;

(c) the respiration and perspiration of the people in the salon.

If the air is too humid, evaporation of perspiration is prevented and the skin's cooling mechanism cannot work effectively. This results in the body overheating, and causes people to feel hot, tired and irritable, and could lead to fainting.

A *wall hygrometer* may be used to measure humidity so that ventilation can be adjusted accordingly. A suitable hair hygrometer is shown in Fig. 6.3.

The working of a hair hygrometer depends on the fact that hair is hygroscopic and increases in length as it absorbs moisture, decreasing in length if it loses moisture. The hygrometer contains a bundle of degreased hairs fixed at one end, with the other end attached through a spring to a pointer which moves over a scale.

As the humidity increases, the hairs absorb moisture, become longer and the pointer moves up the scale. If the humidity decreases, the hairs give up water to the air, become shorter and the pointer moves lower on the scale. The hygrometer measures relative humidity as a percentage.

$$\% \text{ Relative humidity } = \frac{\text{Actual weight of water vapour in any volume of air}}{\substack{\text{Weight of water vapour the air could hold, in the same} \\ \text{volume at the same temperature}}} \times 100$$

The relative humidity should be 50–60 per cent to ensure comfort in the salon.

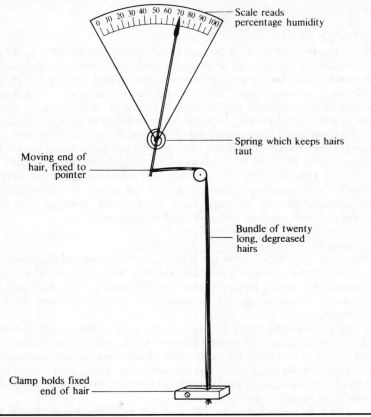

Scale reads percentage humidity

Spring which keeps hairs taut

Moving end of hair, fixed to pointer

Bundle of twenty long, degreased hairs

Clamp holds fixed end of hair

Fig. 6.3 The hair hygrometer

3. The movement of air

If the air is too still, increased local humidity close to the body prevents efficient evaporation of perspiration, leading to overheating. On the other hand, if cold air is moving too quickly people may feel a draught, and the rate of evaporation of moisture from the wet hair of clients may be increased so causing excessive cooling. Ventilation should ensure fresh air without causing a draught. A fan is useful to keep air moving in hot weather.

4. *The purity of the air*

During respiration, oxygen is used up and an increased amount of carbon dioxide is breathed out. Oxygen is also used up during combustion of fuels such as coal, oil and natural gas, and again carbon dioxide is produced. In spite of these changes, the proportion of oxygen and carbon dioxide in fresh air remains constant due to *photosynthesis* in plants (see Fig. 6.4). In this process green plants use carbon dioxide to produce plant food and give out oxygen, though this only takes place if chlorophyll (the green pigment in leaves) and sunlight are present.

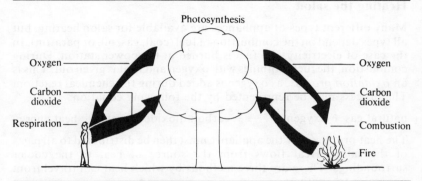

Fig. 6.4 The oxygen-carbon dioxide balance

Photosynthesis may be represented by the following equation:

Carbon dioxide + water + energy from sunlight ——→ oxygen + starch for plant food

However, in a badly ventilated room, there could be a decrease in the amount of oxygen and a corresponding rise in carbon dioxide but the effect would be slight.

The occupants of a salon may be affected by fumes from the chemicals used. Such substances as perm lotions, ammonia and lacquer produce unpleasant smells and may irritate the lining of the nose, throat and lungs. Gases, including unpleasant smells, quickly diffuse or spread to all parts of the salon. Good ventilation ensures that such fumes are quickly removed.

The problem of condensation

Excessive humidity may lead to problems of condensation. As warm moist air cools, it cannot hold as much moisture and the air may become saturated. If further cooling takes place, some of the moisture is deposited as liquid droplets as condensation takes place. This usually occurs if warm moist air comes into contact with cold surfaces such as a cold wall or window, a mirror or cold water pipes. Water is deposited on the surface, causing windows and mirrors to 'steam up', and droplets of water to trickle down the walls.

Condensation may be prevented if water vapour is removed frequently by good ventilation and the various surfaces are kept warm. Heaters may be placed alongside windows or the windows may be double glazed. Walls may be insulated by applying sheets of polystyrene.

Heating the salon

Many different types of appliances are available for salon heating, but all types depend on the combustion of fuel (coal, gas, oil, or paraffin). In the case of electricity, the fuel is burned at the power station. During combustion, the fuel combines with oxygen and heat is given out. This is an *oxidation process*, as oxygen is added during the chemical reaction. The process may be represented by the following equation:

natural gas + oxygen───────> carbon dioxide + water + heat energy

The heat produced by the appliance must then be distributed to all parts of the salon. Heat flows from the source of heat to the cooler surroundings. There are three methods by which heat can travel from one point to another:

1. Conduction
This is the way heat travels through a solid, each molecule passing the heat to the molecule next to it. Some substances are better conductors of heat than others, the best conductors being metals. Substances such as polystyrene, glass fibre, wood, hair and water are poor conductors or good insulators.

Experiment 6.2 To illustrate conduction
Attach several drawing pins to a metal rod by means of wax and support the rod at one end as shown in Fig. 6.5. Heat the unsupported end by a bunsen flame. The pins drop off the rod in turn when the wax melts, proving that the heat is being passed along the bar.

Experiment 6.3. To show that water is a poor conductor of heat
Secure a small piece of ice in a boiling tube by means of a piece of wire to prevent the ice from floating when the tube is filled with cold water. Heat the top of the tube as shown in Fig. 6.6. The water will boil whilst the ice remains intact, indicating that the heat has not been conducted to the bottom of the tube by the water (or by the glass).

2. Convection
Convection is the way in which heat travels through a liquid or a gas by the movement of hot particles.

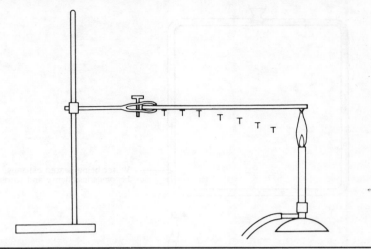

Fig. 6.5 Conduction

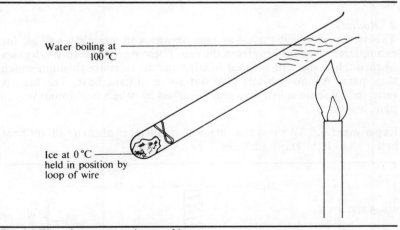

Water boiling at
100 °C

Ice at 0 °C
held in position by
loop of wire

Fig. 6.6 Water is a poor conductor of heat

Experiment 6.4 To demonstrate convection
The circulation of water in the apparatus shown in Fig 6.7 is indicated by
the movement of colour due to potassium permanganate crystals placed
at A. The circulation caused by warmed particles is known as a
convection current.

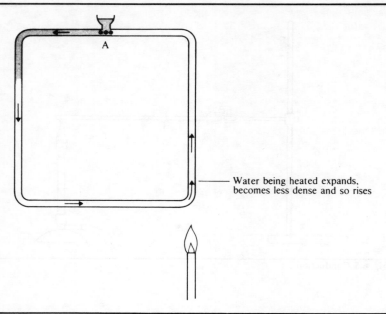

Water being heated expands, becomes less dense and so rises

Fig. 6.7 Convection

3. *Radiation*

This is the way heat travels as rays or waves in straight lines, as, for example, the radiant heat from the sun. These waves pass through gases or through a vacuum without heating the air or space through which they pass. All hot objects give out some radiant heat. The heat is reflected by some substances and absorbed by others in a similar way to light waves.

Experiment 6.5 To show that black matt surfaces absorb radiant heat better than light shiny surfaces

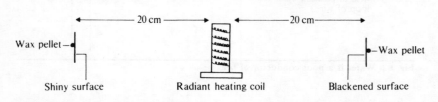

Fig. 6.8 Radiation

Obtain two identical shiny metal plates (or tin lids) and blacken one of them by holding it in a candle flame. Place a few drops of candle wax at the centre back of each plate as shown in Fig. 6.8 and arrange them at equal distances from a radiant heater. Note the time taken for the wax to melt in each case. The wax behind the blackened surface melts first, showing it to be a better absorber of heat. A shiny surface is a good reflector of heat.

Types of heating appliance

The type of heating appliance suitable for a particular salon depends on the size and position of the salon and also on the availability and cost of various fuels. Large salons and those forming part of a large store often have central heating systems which also heat the water for shampooing. Smaller salons may find it more economical to have small fixed or portable heaters.

Central heating systems

1. By circulation of hot water (see Fig. 6.9)

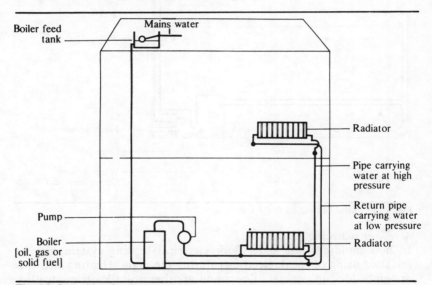

Fig. 6.9 Central heating by hot water

Hot water from a boiler is circulated through narrow bore pipes by an electric pump to radiators, which give out the heat to the room. The term 'radiator' implies transfer of heat by radiation, though most of the heat is transferred to the air and circulates in the rooms by convection. The operating temperature may be controlled by a wall thermostat or a separate thermostat on each radiator. The boiler may also be controlled by a time switch. This type of installation usually provides a supply of hot water for the salon as well. The radiators require wall space which may present difficulties in a salon where much of the equipment is wall based.

2. By ducted air (see Fig. 6.10)
Warm air is circulated through ducts by fans, and enters rooms by grilles near the floor. The electrical system is similar to a large fan-controlled storage heater and uses off-peak electricity. Heat travels round the rooms by convection of hot air.

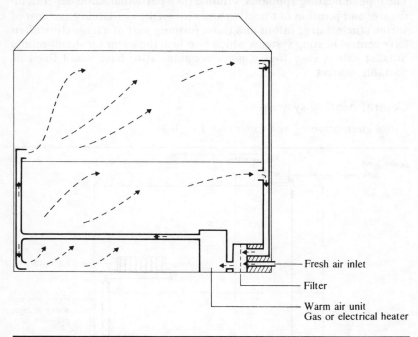

Fresh air inlet

Filter

Warm air unit
Gas or electrical heater

Fig. 6.10 Central heating by ducted warm air

3. Floor warming
In new buildings, an under-floor electrical heating system may be installed using off-peak electricity during the night. Heating elements are embedded in concrete floors and are thermostatically controlled. Since hairdressers are standing all day, they may find this type of heating tiring to the feet.

Other fixed heaters

1. Gas convector heaters with a balanced flue (see Fig. 6.11)
Gas convector heaters are safe for salon use as the flames are entirely enclosed. They are usually connected through an outside wall using a balanced flue. The combustion chamber of the heater is then completely isolated and sealed so that the gases produced during combustion cannot enter the room.

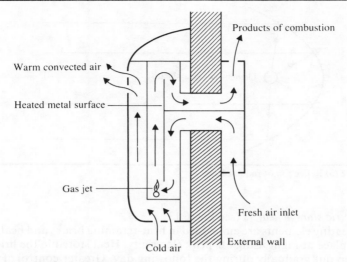

Products of combustion

Warm convected air

Heated metal surface

Gas jet

Fresh air inlet

Cold air

External wall

Fig. 6.11 Gas convector heater with balanced flue

2. Combined radiant and convector gas heaters
Heaters of this type give quick warmth and have a pleasant glow. They may be suitable for a small salon though there is some fire risk unless the radiant elements are well guarded. A flue is always required for gas appliances and may be a balanced flue (see Fig. 6.11) or an open flue, either leading directly to the outside of the building or connected through an existing chimney. The flue carries away the gases produced during combustion. Gas appliances require regular servicing to ensure maximum safety.

3. Wall-mounted radiant electrical heaters (see Fig. 6.12)
This type of heater is safe for salon use, as it has a pull-cord switch and is usually mounted high on the wall. The heating element is enclosed in a silica sheath and the reflector behind the element is pivoted so that the heat can be directed as required.

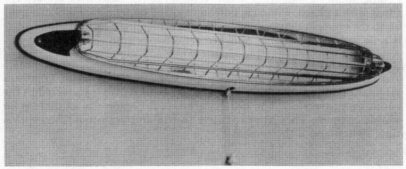

Fig. 6.12 *(a)* Radiant wall-mounted heater

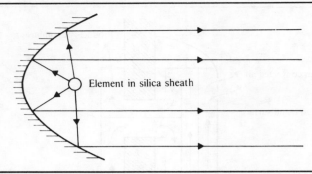

Fig. 6.12 *(b)* Reflection of radiant heat

4. Electric storage heaters (see Fig. 6.13)
The heating elements are embedded in heat-retaining bricks and heating takes place at night using off-peak electricity. Heat stored in the bricks is given out gradually during the following day. Greater control of the heat output is possible if the heaters are fan assisted.

5. Tubular electrical heaters
These heaters give a good background heat but require a considerable amount of wall space, which may be a disadvantage in a salon. A tubular heater placed near the glass of a shop window is useful to reduce condensation.

Portable heaters

Portable electric heaters are useful for local heating of a particular area.

1. Radiant electric fires
This type of heater must be carefully sited if it is not to be a fire hazard. People standing too close are at risk, although such fires are always fitted with a guard. Cut hair, cotton wool, or paper accidently dropped on to the element may cause fire. Heat is transmitted by radiation which is reflected from a highly polished reflector behind the element.

2. Oil-filled radiators
An electrical heating element in the base of the radiator creates a circulation of hot oil within the radiator. Heat is also transferred to the room by convection. The heaters are safe for salon use as there is no visible element. They are expensive to run and are often fitted with a time switch and a thermostat.

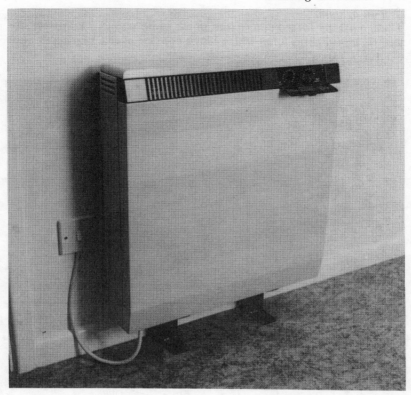

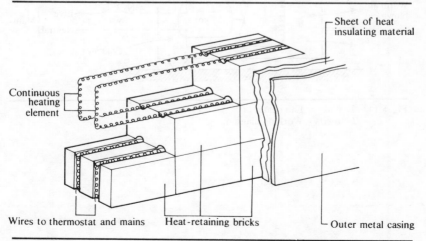

Sheet of heat insulating material

Continuous heating element

Wires to thermostat and mains   Heat-retaining bricks

Outer metal casing

Fig. 6.13 *(Top)*   Storage heater
          (Bottom)   Interior of storage heater

3. Fan heaters

These work by forced convection in the same way as a hairdryer. An electric motor turns a fan which blows cool air over a heating element (see Fig. 6.14).

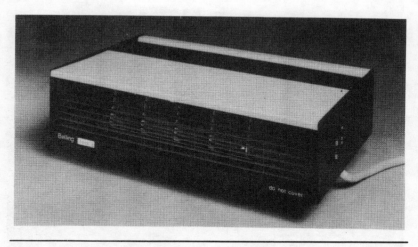

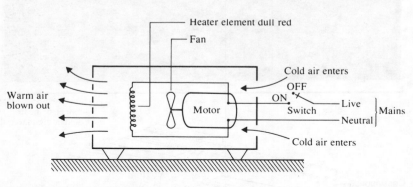

Fig. 6.14 *(Top)*   Fan heater
              (Bottom) Working diagram

4. Convector heaters

Convectors give a good background heat and are safe for salon use as there is no visible element. Convection currents are set up as the air circulates through the appliance (see Fig. 6.15).

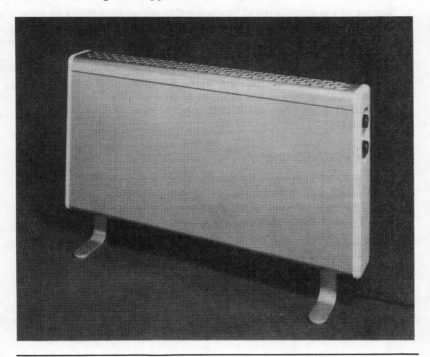

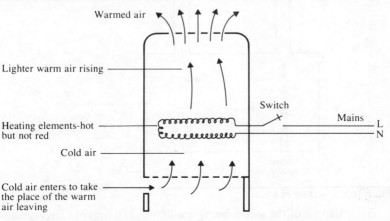

Fig. 6.15 *(Top)*   Convector heater
            (Bottom)   Working diagram

Ventilation of the salon

Good ventilation should replace stale air with fresh air without causing a draught. To ensure this the following conditions should be satisfied:

1. The air in the salon should be changed three or four times an hour.
2. Cool air should not enter the room at floor level as this is draughty to the feet.
3. Air entering the room above head level should be directed upwards so that it is slightly warmed before moving downwards. Clients with wet hair feel a cooling effect due to the evaporation of moisture, and further cooling by a down draught of cool air could be unpleasant.
4. Air outlets should be smaller than inlets so that air does not circulate too quickly.

Methods of ventilation

A salon may be ventilated by natural or artificial means.
Natural ventilation includes the use of windows, doors and ventilating bricks. This type of ventilation depends on convection currents, and may be assisted by the heating appliances in the salon.

Experiment 6.6 To demonstrate convection in a gas
The air heated by the candle flame (see Fig. 6.16) rises and sets up a convection current as shown by the movement of smoke particles.

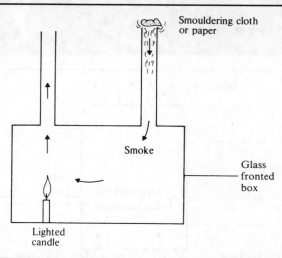

Smouldering cloth or paper

Smoke

Glass fronted box

Lighted candle

Fig. 6.16 Convection in a gas

The warm air of the salon, being less dense than the cold air, rises and may pass out of the room through open windows high on the outside walls or through ventilation bricks. Fresh air enters by windows and doors, though its entry is difficult to control. Draughts may be caused, blowing cut hair about. Dust, smoke or fumes from passing traffic may blow into the salon. Some control is possible by fitting *Cooper's discs* in windows. The inner disc can be rotated so that its openings coincide with similar holes in the window (see Fig. 6.17).

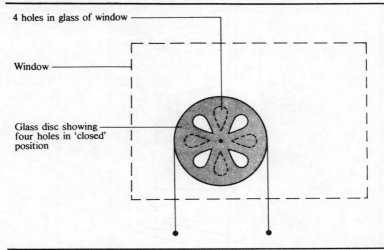

4 holes in glass of window

Window

Glass disc showing four holes in 'closed' position

Fig. 6.17 Cooper's disc

Hopper windows make good inlets as they direct the air upwards on entry (see Fig. 6.18).

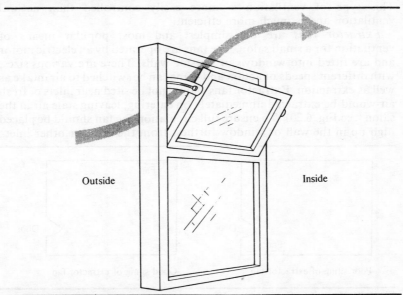

Outside

Inside

Fig. 6.18 A hopper window

Louvred windows consist of movable strips of glass (see Fig. 6.19). They may be used as outlets or inlets of air according to the position of the strips when the louvres are open.

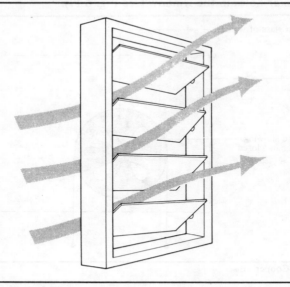

Fig. 6.19 A louvred window

Artificial or assisted ventilation involves the use of mechanical aids. This type of ventilation is more easily controlled than natural ventilation and is much more efficient.

Extractor fans are the simplest and most popular means of ventilation for a small salon. The fans are operated by an electric motor and are fitted into windows or outside walls. There are various sizes, with different speeds of action and some can be switched to air intake as well as extraction. Extractor fans should not be sited near inlets or fresh air would be extracted immediately on entering, leaving stale air in the salon (see Fig. 6.20). To ensure full circulation the fan should be placed high up in the wall or window furthest from the door or other inlet.

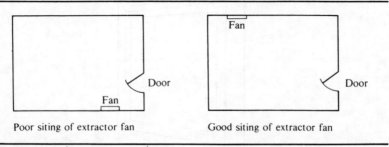

Poor siting of extractor fan   Good siting of extractor fan

Fig. 6.20 The siting of an extractor fan

The number or size of fans can be calculated from manufacturer's data, room size and the number of changes of air required per hour.

Example: Room size $= 8$ m $\times$ 4 m $\times$ 3 m $= 96$ m³ (cubic metres)
Number of air changes required $= 4$ per hour
Therefore, air movement $= 96 \times 4 = 384$ m³ per hour.

A fan removing air at this rate may be chosen from the manufacturer's data.

In large buildings, an *exhaust system* using powerful extractor fans in the roof may withdraw stale air through ducts, and fresh air enters through windows and doors. Alternatively, in the *plenum system*, fresh air is forced into the building by fans, so increasing the air pressure inside and preventing incoming draughts. Any air leakage consists of stale air passing outwards through windows and doors.

The plenum and exhaust systems may be combined to form a *balanced system* in which both intake of fresh air and extraction of stale air are controlled by fans in the roof. A more complicated balanced system in which air is filtered and adjusted to a suitable temperature and humidity is known as *air conditioning* (see Fig. 6.21). Small air conditioning units are available to control the air in a single room. These sometimes recirculate the air after filtering and adjusting the temperature.

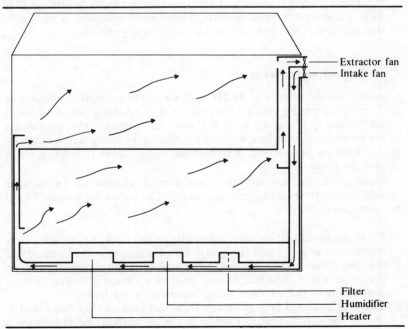

Extractor fan
Intake fan

Filter
Humidifier
Heater

Fig. 6.21 The air conditioning of a building

Ventilation during wig cleaning

Wig cleaning by the use of grease solvents should ideally take place in the open air. If this is impossible, a very well ventilated room is required. Dry cleaning by solvents should not be carried out in the salon nor should these solvents ever be used on the head of a client. Wig-cleaning solvents may be divided into two classes:

1. *Petroleum products* such as hexane, white spirit or naphtha are hydro-carbons so contain only hydrogen and carbon atoms. They are volatile liquids which give off unpleasant though non-toxic fumes. Petroleum solvents are highly flammable and must not be used near naked flames.
2. *Chlorinated hydrocarbons* such as carbon tetrachloride, trichlorethylene and trichloroethane are colourless volatile liquids. They are non-flammable and all have a sweetish smell. Protective gloves should be worn when using these solvents as they are very de-greasing and may cause cracking or blistering of the skin.

   Carbon tetrachloride is now rarely used since it produces a heavy toxic vapour with anaesthetic properties. A person overcome by the fumes and falling to the ground falls into the vapour. A poisonous gas called phosgene is formed if the vapour comes into contact with hot metals or lighted cigarettes. Trichlorethylene is less toxic than carbon tetrachloride but its fumes are anaesthetic and at lower concentrations may cause nausea and vomiting. Trichloroethane is the least toxic of these chlorinated solvents and the fumes are no more hazardous than those of the petroleum solvents. Since trichloroethane is also non-flammable it is now the preferred solvent for wig cleaning.

Clothing for salon wear

Clothing should always be designed to assist the normal regulation of body temperature by keeping the body cool in hot conditions and warm when the surroundings are cold. It should never impede the movements of the wearer, nor interfere with the circulation by being too tight at any point. Ease of laundering is important as hairdressers require clean clothes every day.

Since salons are usually warm and humid, clothes for salon wear should enable the body to lose heat easily. The following points should be considered:

1. Clothing should fit loosely, especially at the neck, to allow an easy circulation of air round the body. This ensures that the humidity of the air close to the skin is kept low, enabling perspiration to evaporate easily. The rate of evaporation is increased by the upward movement of the air after being warmed by the body.
2. The fabric should be a good conductor of heat so that body heat is lost to the surroundings. Cotton is a better conductor of heat than either nylon or wool and so is cooler.

3. The material should allow air to move easily through it and not enmesh air between its fibres. Wool traps air in pockets between the fibres and these form insulation, so that woollen garments are warm. Nylon often has a very close weave and does not allow the passage of air, so nylon keeps the body warm. Cotton is a cool fabric unless it has a special cellular weave designed to trap air pockets.

4. Underclothing which is worn next to the skin must absorb perspiration and then allow it to evaporate at a moderate rate which will cool the skin but not chill it, nor hold the moisture too long so that the garment becomes wet. Cotton is the most suitable fabric as it absorbs well and keeps the body cool. Wool absorbs well but is too warm for salon wear. Nylon has very poor absorbency and is uncomfortable to wear next to the skin.

5. Overalls or outer wear for the salon should be water repellent in case of accidental splashing whilst shampooing. They should also be resistant to dirt, creases and the chemicals used in the salon. Light coloured garments are cooler in sunshine or in radiant heat as the heat is reflected, but pale-coloured nylon tends to discolour easily and holds dirt by electrostatic attraction. Nylon is easy to launder and dries quickly but is uncomfortable to wear as it retains body heat and increases sweating. Rayon is cheaper than cotton and nylon but is not very hard wearing and does not keep its shape well. Cotton can be treated to make it drip dry, and often has polyester fibres blended with it to improve the drying properties and make it easier to iron. Cotton/polyester overalls are cool and comfortable to wear though they need more laundering than nylon.

Questions

1. Explain the following statements.
   (a) the skin goes white or blue with cold;
   (b) the skin becomes red after strenuous exercise;
   (c) a tight-fitting metallic screw-cap on a glass bottle may be eased by placing the cap under hot water;
   (d) wig-cleaning solvents should never be used on a client's head.

2. What is meant by (a) evaporation and (b) boiling? What are the main differences between the two?

3. Heat may travel by conduction, convection or radiation. Explain each step in the process as heat travels from each of the following.
   (a) the surface of the skin to the surroundings during cooling of the body;
   (b) the heated bars of a heat perm machine to the clips;
   (c) a hair dryer to a client's head;
   (d) the element of an electric storage heater to the air in a salon;
   (e) the element in an oil-filled electric radiator to the air of a salon;
   (f) an electric light bulb to a person standing below.

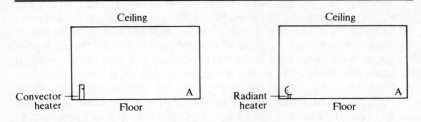

Fig. 6.22 Question 3

4. Figure 6.22 shows the side view of two salons, one heated by a convector heater and the other by a radiant heater. On each diagram, show by the use of arrows how the heat reaches the person at A.

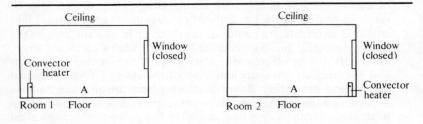

Fig. 6.23 Question 4

5. Figure 6.23 shows the side views of two salons heated by convector heaters. Show, by means of arrows on the diagrams, the direction of the circulation of warm air in the two rooms. In which room would a person at A feel more comfortable? Give a reason for your choice.

Chapter 7

The salon electricity supply

Many salon appliances are powered by electricity, and a basic understanding of electrical circuits and electric current helps to ensure the safe and efficient handling of these appliances. Simple electrical repairs such as re-wiring plugs and replacing fuses may save the hairdresser considerable time and expense.

What is electricity?

If a nylon brush is used on dry, newly washed hair, the hairs spring apart, tend to cling to the brush and follow its movements. The hair is difficult to manage because it has become charged with electricity. The production of this electrical charge is explained by studying the structure of atoms.

All atoms are made up of two different types of electrically charged particles. Positively charged particles, called *protons*, lie in the nucleus of the atom and negatively charged particles, called *electrons*, move in orbit round the nucleus. Each atom thus resembles a miniature solar system (see Fig. 7.1).

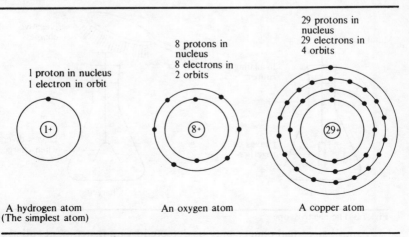

29 protons in nucleus
29 electrons in 4 orbits

8 protons in nucleus
8 electrons in 2 orbits

1 proton in nucleus
1 electron in orbit

A hydrogen atom
(The simplest atom)

An oxygen atom

A copper atom

Fig. 7.1 The structure of atoms

The atoms of each different element have a different number of circulating electrons, but each atom is electrically neutral because the number of negatively charged orbital electrons is balanced by an equal number of positively charged protons in the nucleus. Electrons are much lighter than protons and are more easily removed from the atom.

The friction of rubbing a brush along the hair removes electrons from atoms in the hair. These electrons collect on the brush, giving it a negative charge. Loss of electrons leaves the hair positively charged. Since like charges repel each other and opposite charges attract each other, the hairs fly apart but are attracted to the brush (see Fig. 7.2). The electrical charges on the brush and hair are known as *static electricity* because the electricity is stationary, or sometimes as *frictional electricity* because the electricity is produced by friction between two substances.

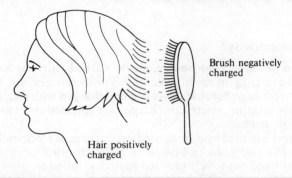

Brush negatively charged

Hair positively charged

Fig. 7.2 Static electricity

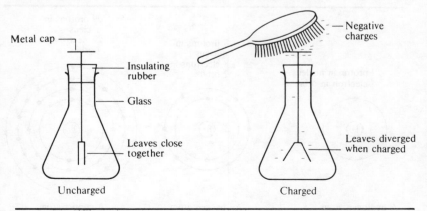

Metal cap

Insulating rubber

Glass

Leaves close together

Uncharged

Negative charges

Leaves diverged when charged

Charged

Fig. 7.3 The electroscope

A small electrical charge may be detected by an instrument called *an electroscope*. If the charged brush is brought into contact with the cap of an electroscope, the electrical charges travel down the rod to the gold leaves which spring apart because the like charges on them repel each other (see Fig. 7.3).

When electrons move through a substance they form a flow called an *electric current* (see Fig. 7.4).

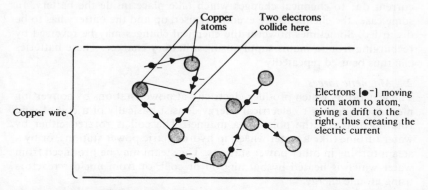

Fig. 7.4 An electric current in a copper wire

Conductors and insulators

The outer electrons of some elements, especially metal elements, are only loosely held in the atoms and these electrons can easily be detached and made to pass from atom to atom through the substance. Such substances are said to be *good conductors* of electricity as electricity flows easily through them.

In substances like nylon and rubber, where the electrons are more firmly held, it is difficult to make an electric current flow. Such substances are called electrical *insulators* (see Table 7.1). Copper wires, being good conductors and much cheaper than silver, are used to carry the electric current in domestic wiring. The wires are surrounded by an insulating layer of plastic or rubber to contain the current in the wiring.

Table 7.1 Conductors and insulators

Good conductors	Insulators
Silver (best)	Rubber
Copper (very good)	Nylon
Aluminium	Plastic
Most other metals	Air
	Porcelain
	Glass
	Dry hair

Sources of electric current

An electric current may be produced by:

1. Chemical reactions

Batteries such as those used in torches and portable radios produce a current due to chemical changes which take place inside the battery. In some cases the chemicals are eventually used up and the battery has to be discarded. Sometimes however the chemical changes may be reversed by recharging from a mains supply using a battery charger. These batteries can thus be used repeatedly.

2. Magnetic forces

The generators which produce electricity at power stations by converting mechanical energy to electrical energy consist basically of a coil of wire rotating between the poles of a magnet. The coil is rotated either by water turbine (like a water wheel) in hydroelectric power stations, or by a steam turbine in other power stations. The steam may be produced from water which is heated by burning oil or coal, or from nuclear reactors using atomic energy.

Circuits

An electric current will only flow if there is a complete conducting pathway from the source of electricity (the battery or generator), through an appliance and back again to the source. This pathway is called a *circuit*. A switch is used to complete or to break the circuit and thus to start and stop the flow of electricity (see Fig. 7.5).

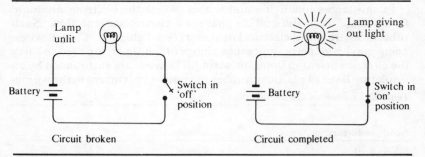

Fig. 7.5 Electrical circuits

The distribution of mains electricity

Mains electricity is carried from the power generating station along overhead cables held by pylons, and finally enters the buildings of a town by underground cables (see Fig. 7.6). The circuit from the generator is shown in Fig. 7.6. This circuit is completed when an appliance is plugged into a socket and switched on. The current leaving the power station travels to the salon along a feed cable or live wire. It returns to the power station along a neutral or return wire. Switches should always be installed in the live or feed wire. If possible examine a discarded switch to see the method of operation. In the 'off' position an air gap is created in the circuit and the current cannot pass.

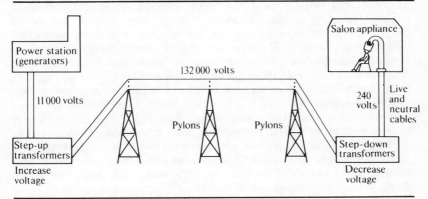

Fig. 7.6 The distribution of electricity

Voltage or electrical pressure

A battery or a mains generator acts like a pump which drives the electricity through the wiring. The electrical pressure produced by the battery or generator is known as its *voltage* and is measured in units called *volts*. A battery produces only a low voltage and is incapable of operating a salon hair dryer or an electric fire, but is suitable for lighting a torch bulb or working a radio. The voltage produced by a generator is usually 11 000 volts. This is increased before passing over the pylons and decreased to 240 volts before reaching a house or salon (see Fig. 7.6). Typical voltages are shown in Table 7.2.

Table 7.2   Voltage

Small torch battery	1·5	volts
Transistor radio battery		
(6 cell)	9	volts
Car battery	12	volts
Mains generator	11 000	volts
reduced to	240	volts for a domestic supply
or to	110	volts for the domestic supply in some foreign countries

It is important that appliances are used at the correct voltage. Foreign appliances designed to be used at 110 volts will be damaged if plugged into a 240 volt supply. Electric shavers are sometimes designed to work at either 110 or 240 volts by the operation of a switch.

Salon circuits

The electrical installation for a salon consists of several individual circuits including a lighting circuit, one or more circuits for power plugs, and often separate circuits for immersion heaters or instantaneous water heaters. These circuits radiate from a central distribution box or *consumer unit* which contains the *main switch* and the *main fuses* for each circuit. In older distributive type installations (see Fig. 7.7), there may be a number of separate switches and fuse boxes as each power socket was separately wired to a fuse box. Modern installations are based on ring main circuits for power sockets (see Fig. 7.8). Electric storage heaters and water heaters, which are time controlled to operate only during cheap night rate periods, are connected to a separate consumer unit and fitted with a time switch. The consumer unit is usually placed near to the *meter* and the Electricity Board's *sealed fuse box*. The sealed fuse box must only be opened by the Board's engineers.

The distributive installation (see Fig. 7.7)

In this system:
1. There are often two or more different sizes of socket and therefore plugs of several sizes are required.
2. The cost of installation is greater than for ring main circuits.
3. The addition of new sockets is expensive as each is wired separately to the fuse box.
4. There are no fuses in the plugs.

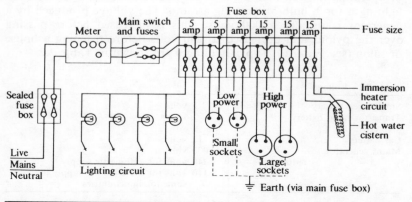

Fig. 7.7 The distributive circuit (older type)

Modern installation (see Fig. 7.8)

In ring main circuits:

1. The circuit cable goes from room to room round the salon in a closed loop to which sockets may be wired at any point.
2. All the sockets are the same size and are designed to take standard 13 amp three-pin plugs, so that any appliance may be plugged into any socket.
3. Less wiring is required than for a distributive installation.
4. It is easier and cheaper to add extra sockets.
5. Each plug has a fuse which is adjusted in size to suit the power of the appliance to which it is attached.

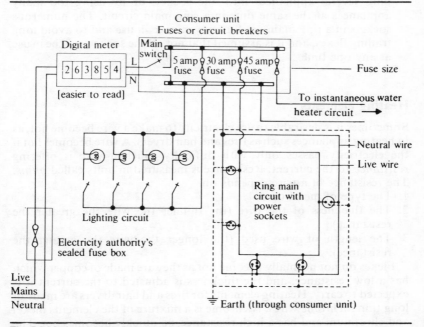

Fig. 7.8 Modern installation with ring main circuit

Salon wiring and the overloading of circuits

The wiring in a salon lies mainly behind the plaster or under the floor boards, though in modern installations it may be fitted in plastic channels or trunking laid at skirting level over the wall plaster, thus allowing easy access for later modifications. The only visible parts of the circuits are the socket outlets and the switches. Insulated copper wire is used for the circuit wiring and also for the flexes attached to appliances. The thickness of the wire varies in different circuits and also in the flexes of different appliances. The thicker the wire the more current it can safely carry without becoming hot. If a cable carries a greater current than that for which it was designed it is *overloaded*. It will become hot and may start a fire. Overloading should cause the circuit fuse to melt, so safely cutting off the current.

The size of the current flowing in a conductor is measured in units called *amperes* (A or amps). The thick cable of an electric cooker or instantaneous water heater is designed to carry a current of up to 30 amps but that of a lighting circuit only 5 amps.

A circuit may be overloaded by:
1. Connecting heating appliances to a lighting circuit.
2. Plugging too many appliances into a circuit by using an adaptor to plug several appliances into one socket, or by using too many appliances at the same time in a ring main circuit. The numerous sockets in a ring main are for convenience in use and to avoid long trailing flexes, and it is assumed that not all the sockets will be in use at any one time.

Heating elements

Sometimes it is desirable to use electricity to make a wire become hot, as in heating appliances such as fires and hair dryers. A wire becomes hot if the electricity passes only with difficulty. Such a wire is offering *resistance* to the current. Resistance is measured in units called *ohms*. The resistance of a wire depends on:
1. The type of metal used.
2. The thickness of the wire (the thinner the wire the greater the resistance).
3. The length of wire used (the longer the wire the greater the resistance).

Flexes do not normally become hot as they are made of copper which has a low resistance, and the thickness is adjusted to the current it is expected to carry. Heating elements for fires and hair dryers are made of long thin *nichrome* wires. Nichrome is a mixture of the elements nickel and chromium and has a high resistance, so quickly becomes hot. The filaments of electric light bulbs are made of high resistance *tungsten* which becomes so hot that it gives out light as well as heat.

Experiment 7.1. To show the heating effect of a current
The apparatus shown in Fig. 7.9 may be used to vary the size of the current flowing through a nichrome wire. Gradually increase the current, by starting with the resistance at its maximum and decreasing it step by step. The temperature of the wire may be roughly noted by touch, by placing a small paper 'rider' on the wire and then by noting colour changes. Observations such as warm, very warm, hot, chars paper, dull red, bright red, orange, white, melts, can be made as the current increases. If the nichrome wire does not become hot, repeat with

a shorter length. Repeat the experiment by replacing the nichrome wire with copper wire and then with fuse wire (2 amp).

Record the results thus:

Current	Effect on nichrome	Effect on copper	Effect on fuse wire

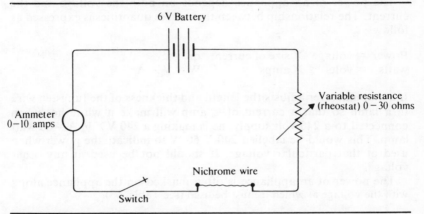

Fig. 7.9 The heating effect of a current

The results show that the heat produced in a wire increases as the current increases.

The size of the current and Ohm's Law

The size of the current (amps) flowing through a conductor depends on:
1. The resistance of the wire (ohms).
2. The electrical pressure (volts).
The relationship between these quantities is:

$$\text{Size of current} = \frac{\text{electrical pressure}}{\text{resistance}} \quad \text{or}$$

$$\text{amps} = \frac{\text{volts}}{\text{ohms}}$$

This is known as *Ohm's Law*. Calculations involving this law are made during the design of appliances. For example, calculations are made to find the length and thickness of the tungsten wire required in making a light bulb of a particular power.

The power of an appliance

The power of an appliance is measured in *watts* and is the rate at which the appliance uses electrical energy. A high powered light bulb of 250 watts will give a bright light; a low powered bulb of 15 watts will give a dim light only suitable for decorative purposes. The higher the wattage of the appliance the greater the consumption of electricity.

The power of an appliance depends on both the voltage and the current. The relationship between these three quantities is expressed as follows:

Power = voltage × size of current   or
watts = volts   × amps $W = V \times A$

If a manufacturer adjusts the length and thickness of the tungsten wire in a lamp so that a current of $\frac{1}{4}$ amp will make it white hot when connected to a 240 volt supply, he is making a 240 V × $\frac{1}{4}$ A = 60 watt lamp. This would be labelled 240 V 60 W to indicate the power when used at that particular voltage. It should not be used at any other voltage.

The power of an appliance is often marked on the appliance along with the voltage at which it must be used (see Table 7.3).

Table 7.3   The typical wattage of appliances

Hair clippers	20 W
Extractor fan	25 W
Marcel iron heater	250 W
Hand hair dryer	500 W
Salon hair dryer	1000–1500 W
Steamer	750 W
Washing machine without heater	300 W
Washing machine with heater	3000 W
Immersion heater	3000 W
Instantaneous water heater	3 – 9 kW

(1000 watts = 1 kilowatt or 1 kW)

Fuses

The consumer unit contains a *fuse* for each circuit and, in addition, appliances often have fused plugs and sometimes fused switches. A fuse is a safety device to stop the flow of electricity if the current becomes greater than the wiring can carry without overheating. The fuse wire is designed to be the weakest part of the circuit and will not carry as much current as the wiring it protects. When the current exceeds the safety limit the fuse wire becomes hot, melts and cuts off the current. It thus protects the wiring and the appliance from over-heating and prevents a possible outbreak of fire. The fuse always forms part of the live wire of the circuit.

Circuit fuses (main fuses in the consumer unit)

Each circuit fuse has a different rating (in amps) depending on the maximum size of current the circuit is required to carry. A lighting circuit contains a very fine fuse wire with a current rating of 5A, so that the fuse would melt if the current exceeded 5 amps. A ring circuit has a thicker fuse wire with a current rating of 30 A. The current ratings for different circuits are shown in Table 7.4.

Table 7.4 The current rating for different circuits

Circuit	Current rating of fuse wire in amps	Colour of cartridge or spot on holder
Lighting	5 A	White
Immersion heater	15 A	Blue
Storage heater	20 A	Yellow
Ring main	30 A	Red
Instantaneous water heater	45 A	Green

The circuit fuse may melt or 'blow' due to:
1. Overloading the circuit.
2. Faulty wiring. Worn insulation could lead to a *short circuit* when the live and neutral wires touch, as the appliance is by-passed causing a large surge of current. Short circuits may also result from piercing cables whilst driving nails into floor boards or walls, and from dislodging wires from the terminal screws of plugs by pulling the flex.
3. A faulty appliance causing a short circuit. If the appliance plug is correctly fused, this fuse should melt and not the circuit fuse.
4. Old or corroded fuse wire.

Types of circuit fuse
There are two types of circuit fuse:

1. Rewirable fuses
These are made of tinned copper. The fuse wire is held in a ceramic carrier or tube attached to a plastic fuse holder, and is secured by two screws. Each fuse holder is colour coded with a spot of colour which indicates the size of fuse to be used in that holder. The colour spots are listed in Table 7.4.

2. Cartridge fuses
These consist of a fuse wire contained in a small ceramic tube and attached to metal caps at each end of the fuse (see Fig. 7.10). The tube also contains sand in case sparking occurs when the fuse blows. The cartridge fits into a metal or plastic clamp in a fuse holder. Cartridges have the same current ratings as rewirable fuses and this is stamped on the cartridge. The colour of the cartridge varies, and corresponds to the

spot of colour on the fuse holder (see Table 7.4). It is impossible to fit the wrong size of cartridge into a holder as they differ in physical size; the higher the current rating, the larger the cartridge.

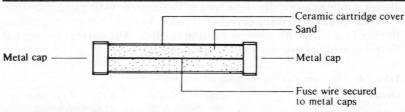

Ceramic cartridge cover
Sand
Metal cap
Metal cap
Fuse wire secured to metal caps

Fig. 7.10 A cartridge fuse

Plug fuses

Plug fuses are cartridge type fuses designed to protect an individual appliance and its flexible cord from damage by overheating, due to a fault in either the flex or the appliance. All plug cartridge fuses have the same physical size but are available in three current ratings as follows:
1. 3 A current rating for use with appliances up to 720 watts.
2. 5 A current rating for use with appliances of 720–1200 watts.
3. 13 A current rating for use with appliances with a loading of between 1200 and 3000 watts.

Replacing a blown fuse

A blown fuse indicates either overloading or a faulty appliance or faulty wiring. Any fault should be located and corrected or the fuse may blow again as soon as it is replaced.

A card of fuse wires of different ratings or a supply of new cartridges should be kept near the consumer unit in readiness to replace a blown fuse. Time can be saved if the various circuits are labelled inside the consumer unit.

To repair a circuit fuse, disconnect all appliances, switch off the main switch, open the consumer unit and locate the blown fuse by removing the appropriate holder. Remove the cartridge or the old fuse wire. If a rewirable type, thread the new fuse wire through the ceramic holder and tighten the screws, being careful not to stretch the wire when tightening the second screw. Cut off any spare wire. It is important to use the correct size of fuse wire for if the current rating is too high the cables would overheat before the fuse melted. If the fuse is a cartridge type, discard the old fuse and replace with a new one of the same size. Replace the fuse holder, and switch on the main switch.

To replace a plug fuse, unscrew the plug cap, remove and discard the old fuse. Select a new fuse of the correct current rating, insert it in the plug and replace the plug cap.

To calculate the correct size of plug fuse

Examine the wattage plate of the appliance or the manufacturer's leaflet to find the wattage of the appliance and the voltage at which it must be used. Consult an electrician if the voltage is not 240 V. Calculate the size of current which will flow when the appliance is plugged into the 240 V. supply.

$$\text{Since watts} = \text{volts} \times \text{amps}$$
$$\text{size of current (amps)} = \frac{\text{watts}}{\text{volts}}$$

The fuse size must be greater than the size of the normal current, and have a current rating of either 3 A, 5 A or 13 A.

Example: Calculate the correct size of plug fuse for a 1000 W hair dryer on a 240 V supply

$$\text{Size of current through fuse} = \frac{\text{watts}}{\text{volts}} = \frac{1000}{240} = 4 \cdot 2 \text{ amps}$$

A 3 A fuse would be too small, a 5 A fuse is required.

To find the range of wattage permissible with a given fuse

(a) With a 3 amp fuse. (Mains voltage = 240 volts.)
   Maximum current = 3 amps.
   Therefore maximum wattage = volts × amps = 240 × 3 = 720 watts
   Thus a 3 A fuse is used for appliances with a wattage up to 720 W.
(b) With a 5 A fuse.
   Maximum current = 5 amps.
   Maximum wattage = volts × amps = 240 × 5 = 1200 watts.
   Thus a 5 A fuse is used for appliances of 720 − 1200 watts.
(c) With a 13 amp fuse.
   Maximum current = 13 amps
   Maximum wattage = V × A = 240 × 13 = 3120 watts
   Thus a 13 amp fuse is used for appliances of 1200 W − 3120 W
   Appliances with a wattage of over 3000 W, such as instantaneous water heaters (3–9 kW), are wired separately directly to the consumer unit and are not included in a ring main circuit. They would be fitted with a 30 A or 45 A fuse in the consumer unit.

To calculate overloading

Example: If a 1000 W blow dryer and a 250 W light bulb are used in a lighting circuit with a 5 A fuse is the circuit overloaded?
Main voltage = 240 V

$$\text{Size of current} = \frac{\text{wattage of appliances}}{\text{voltage}} = \frac{1000 + 250}{240} = 5 \cdot 2 \text{ amps}$$

Since the current is greater than the fuse size, the circuit is overloaded.

Circuit breakers

In some modern electrical installations the consumer unit contains circuit breakers instead of fuses (see Fig. 7.11). The circuit breaker is an automatic switch which cuts off the supply whenever excess current flows through the circuit, due either to a fault or overloading. The current can be restored simply by switching to the 'on' position when the overload has been cleared or the faulty appliance removed. This is much quicker than replacing a fuse and the installation of circuit breakers is very advantageous in a busy salon.

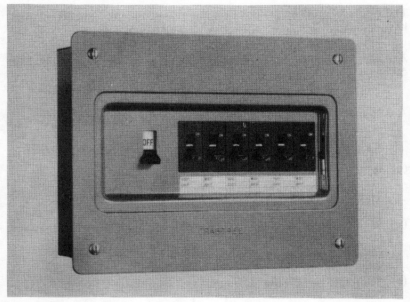

Fig. 7.11 Circuit breakers

The consumer unit may also be fitted with a residual current device or current operated earth-leakage circuit breaker which immediately cuts off the power supply on detecting any leakage of current to earth. It is thus a safeguard against electric shock and fire due to electrical faults.

Plugs and earthing

Electricity may be regarded as being brought to an appliance by the live wire and leaving by the neutral wire. Many appliances have a three-core flex with an *earth wire* in addition to the live and neutral wires. The earth wire connects the outer metal case of an appliance to the earth (the ground). The earth wire must be continuous from the outer metal of the appliance, through the flex, through the plug and socket, along the circuit cable and into the ground under the building, where it is connected to the metal sheath of the Electricity Board's cable (see Fig. 7.12). The earth wire is a safety device designed to prevent electric shock if a fault develops in the appliance. In normal working there is no current flowing through the earth wire.

The three cores of a flex are coated with different coloured plastic insulation so that it is easy to connect the correct wire to the corresponding terminal of the plug. The international colour code for the cores is as follows:

Brown to be connected to the terminal marked live or L.
Blue to be connected to the terminal marked neutral or N.
Green and yellow to be connected to the terminal marked earth, E or I̲

The flex in appliances purchased before 1970 may have the former standard colours:
live – red
neutral – black
earth – green

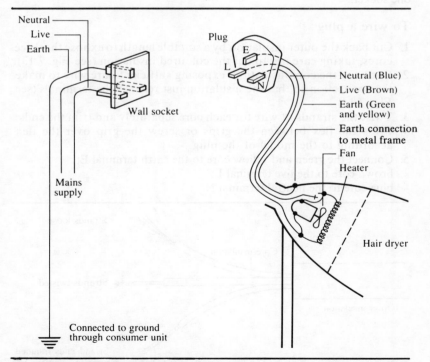

Fig. 7.12 The wiring of a plug and socket

Wrong connections in the plug are dangerous. If the earth wire is attached to the live terminal, the metal frame of the appliance would be live. If the live and neutral wire are interchanged the switch of the appliance would be in the neutral wire and the equipment would be live even when switched off. If foreign appliances have different coloured core insulation, the advice of an electrician should be sought before connecting the plug.

Sockets are often *shuttered* so that the holes are safely covered when not in use. The earth pin which is always longer than the live and neutral pins opens the shutters as the plug is inserted into the socket. The long earth pin also ensures that the appliance is already earthed when the live and neutral pins complete the electrical circuit. The shutters close when the plug is withdrawn. In some modern plugs the live and neutral pins are insulated except at their tips to lessen the possibility of electric shock through touching the pins when inserting or removing the plug.

A plug with damaged or bent pins may not fit the socket perfectly and may become hot if a spark jumps across any small air gap between plug and socket. Such a plug should be replaced as there is danger of fire. Sockets are only intended to carry a current of up to 13 A and may be overloaded if an adaptor is used and several appliances are plugged into one socket.

To wire a plug

1. Cut back the outer insulation by a suitable length to expose the three cores, taking care not to cut the coloured insulation (see Fig. 7.13).
2. Cut back the core insulation, exposing sufficient bare wire to make the connection so that the insulation just reaches the terminals (see Fig. 7.14).
3. Twist the strands of wire for each core separately and trim the ends.
4. Press the flex between the grips or screw the grip over the flex according to the model of the plug.
5. Connect the green and yellow core to the earth terminal E;
   brown core to the live terminal L;
   blue core to the neutral terminal N.

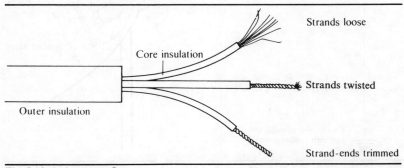

Fig. 7.13 A three-core flex

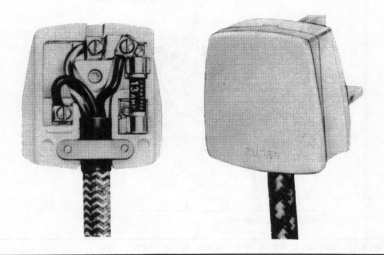

Fig. 7.14 Fused plug

If the wire passes round a screw it should do so in a clockwise direction so that it will stay close to the screw-thread. The insulation should just reach the screw in each case and the screws should be tight.

6. Replace the cartridge fuse checking that it is the correct size for the appliance.
7. Screw down the plug top.

Electric shock

If a person's body completes a mains circuit, the person will experience an electric shock. The effect of the shock will vary according to the size of the current flowing and on the pathway of the current through the body. A small current may produce a tingling feeling, whilst stronger currents may cause contraction of the muscles and burns. Contraction of the muscles in the arms often prevents the release of the person's grip on the appliance. If the current causes contraction of the heart muscles, the heart may stop beating. Breathing will stop if the diaphragm and intercostal muscles between the ribs are contracted. Immediate first aid is required in both cases and is discussed in Chapter 19.

A person may complete a circuit in several different ways:

1. By touching both live and neutral wires (see Fig. 7.15)

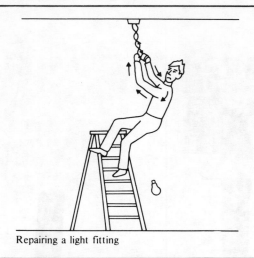

Repairing a light fitting

Fig. 7.15 Effect of touching both live and neutral wires

2. By touching a live wire and an earthed metal

The earth behaves as an electrical conductor. Metal water pipes which enter the ground provide a path to earth. A person in contact with a live wire and a tap or water pipe, may complete a circuit and receive a shock. Touching a plug with wet hands has the same effect as touching a live wire since impure water is a good conductor. If an earthed metal is touched at the same time, a shock will result (see Fig. 7.16).

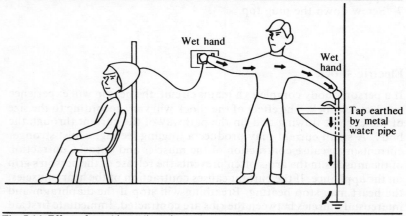

Wet hand

Wet hand

Tap earthed
by metal
water pipe

Fig. 7.16 Effect of touching a live wire and earth

3. By touching a live wire or a live unearthed metal, and the earth

If the outer metal casing of an appliance becomes live due to a fault, and the metal is not earthed, a person can complete the circuit through the ground (see Fig. 7.17). Similarly a person may conduct a current to earth on touching a live wire.

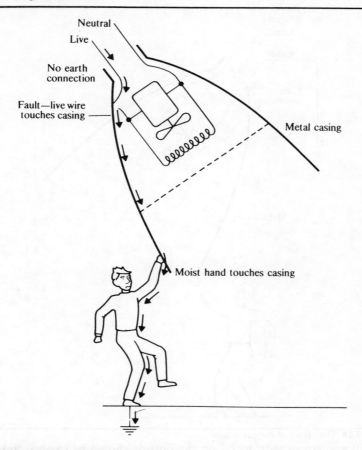

Neutral

Live

No earth connection

Fault—live wire touches casing

Metal casing

Moist hand touches casing

Fig. 7.17 Touching an unearthed metal

The prevention of electric shock

1. By use of an earth wire

If a fault in an appliance with a metal outer casing causes the metal to become live and the metal is correctly earthed, the current is carried safely to earth along the earth wire. The current takes the easiest path to earth and since a person's body would offer a greater resistance to the current than that offered by the metal earth wire, most of the current travels along the earth wire. The low resistance of the earth wire would result in a large surge of current, causing the fuse to melt and the current to be cut off. Thus the earth wire prevents electric shock both by carrying the current to earth, and by ensuring that the fuse will blow (see Fig. 7.18).

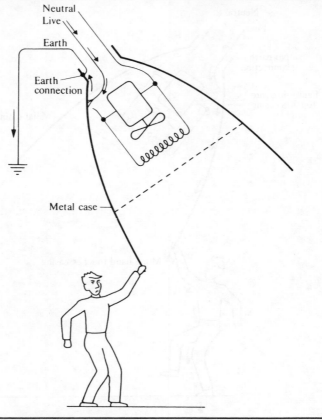

Fig. 7.18 The effect of the earth wire

All appliances with metal on the outside should be earthed unless they bear the sign 🔲 indicating that they are double insulated. In this case the metal is insulated so that there is no danger of a fault causing the outside casing to become live.

2. The use of insulation

Non-conductors such as plastic or rubber are used as insulation against electric shock. The outer covers of switches, plugs and sockets are usually plastic. Flexes are covered with an outer plastic or rubber sheath enclosing the plastic covered cores. The body work of some appliances including some hair dryers is all-insulated by being made entirely of plastic.

Care should be taken to replace worn insulation and broken or cracked plugs and switches. The use of insulation tape should be restricted to temporary repairs and flexes with worn insulation should be replaced. Water may by-pass insulation and an electric shock may result from touching electrical equipment with wet hands.

Costing and the reading of the meter

The size of an electricity bill depends on:
1. The number of units of electricity used.
2. The cost per unit (plus any fixed quarterly charge).

The number of units used is recorded on the electricity meter, and depends on the power (wattage) of the appliances used and the length of time (hours) that the appliances are switched on. The meter multiplies the power (in kilowatts) by the time (in hours) and so records 'units' or *kilowatt hours*.

A 1 kilowatt appliance used for 1 hour uses 1 unit of electricity. Or 1 unit = 1 kilowatt hour (1 kWh).

The cost of electricity varies in different parts of the country. Various tariffs are available for domestic and industrial premises and these should be studied to find the most advantageous.

There may be:
1. A *flat rate* in which each unit is charged at a standard rate.
2. A *quarterly fixed charge* and a standard price per unit.
3. A *block tariff* where a primary block of units is charged at a high rate and the remaining units at the standard rate.
4. An *off-peak tariff* where electricity only used at night for storage heaters and water heaters, is charged at a low rate and separately metered.

To calculate the cost of using appliances

The cost of using an appliance = power of appliance (kW) × hours × cost per unit.

Example (1): What is the cost of using a 2000-watt fire for 8 hours at a cost of 6p a unit?

$$\text{Cost} = \frac{2000}{1000} \times 8 \times 6 = 96\text{p}$$

Example (2): Find the total cost per day of using the following appliances for the times stated. Cost per unit = 5p.

Hair dryer (750 W) used for 6 hours a day.	$\text{Cost} = \frac{750}{1000} \times 6 \times 5 = 22.5\text{p}$
Lights (500 W) used for 10 hours a day.	$\text{Cost} = \frac{500}{1000} \times 10 \times 5 = 25.0\text{p}$
Water heater (2 kW) used 8 hours a day.	$\text{Cost} = \quad 2 \times 8 \times 5 = 80.0\text{p}$
Radio (50 W) used for 10 hours a day.	$\text{Cost} = \frac{50}{1000} \times 10 \times 5 = 2.5\text{p}$
	Total cost per day = 130.0p

Reading the meter

The modern meter is a digital meter and the number of units is read directly. Older meters have a series of dials (see Fig. 7.19). The small dial marked $\frac{1}{10}$ kWh should be ignored as it is used only when testing the meter. Note that the dials are numbered alternately in opposite directions (clockwise, then anticlockwise). When the pointer stands between two numbers read the lowest, except between 0 and 9 when the reading is 9. Meters are usually read every quarter by the Electricity Board's meter reader. The consumption for the quarter is obtained by subtracting the previous reading from the present reading.

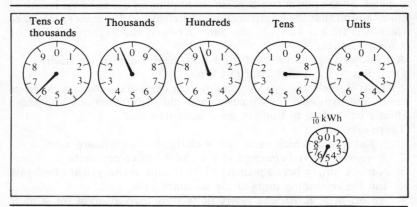

Fig. 7.19 An electricity meter recording 60973·5 units

Calculation of cost per quarter (see fig. 7.20)

Units used between January and April = 66397 — 64382 = 2015 units.
Cost at 5p per unit = 2015 × 5 = £100.75.

State of meter on 1 January: reading 64382

State of meter on 1 April: reading 66397

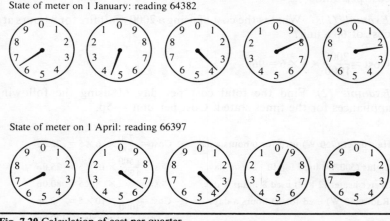

Fig. 7.20 Calculation of cost per quarter

Questions

1. Explain the danger of:
   (a) placing flexes under carpets;   (b) pulling out a plug by the flex;   (c) using electrical appliances with wet hands;   (d) using long trailing flexes.
2. Explain the figures 240 V and 450 W on the plate of a blow-dryer. Calculate the correct size of cartridge fuse required in the plug.
3. A hair dryer is switched on but fails to operate. Suggest possible reasons for the failure. What steps would you take to deal with the situation?
4. You have purchased a foreign electrical appliance. What observations would you make before fitting a plug and using the appliance?
5. (a) Calculate the cost of using a 3 kW immersion heater for 6 hours. Cost per unit is 5p;
   (b) For how long could you use the immersion heater before one unit of electricity had been consumed?

Salon lighting

The aim of salon lighting is to provide sufficient illumination when natural daylight is inadequate. Good well-diffused general lighting should be provided, with additional localised lighting in working areas such as over dressing tables. To avoid eye strain, artificial lighting should not produce an unpleasant glare, nor should there be too much contrast between well lit parts of a room and areas of shadow. The colour of the artificial light should be as near as possible to that of daylight to avoid difficulty in colour matching.

What colour is daylight?

If a narrow beam of sunlight is passed through a triangular glass prism (see Fig. 8.1), the light may be split up or *dispersed* into a band of colour known as a *spectrum* which consists of the seven colours: red, orange, yellow, green, blue, indigo and violet. Indigo is now often omitted as it is hard to distinguish it from violet.

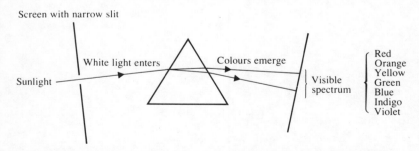

Fig. 8.1 Dispersion

By placing a second identical prism alongside the first prism as shown in Fig. 8.2, the coloured band can be recombined to form white light. Thus sunlight or day light is referred to as *'white light'*, and consists of a mixture of seven colours of light in the proportion produced in its spectrum. Ideally, artificial light should produce the same mixture of colours as sunlight so that objects appear to be the same colour when viewed in either type of light. In practice this is rarely achieved, and hair colouring should therefore be carried out in daylight if possible.

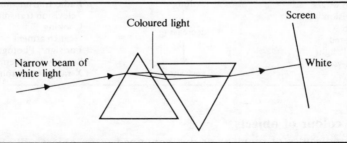

Fig. 8.2 Re-forming white light

Energy waves

In addition to 'visible' white light, sunlight also contains 'invisible' waves called infra-red rays and ultra-violet rays. These together with others such as radiowaves, television waves and X-rays, form a series of energy waves called *electromagnetic waves*. The various waves differ from each other because of their different *wavelengths*, a wavelength being the distance between two adjacent crests of a wave-train (see Fig. 8.3).

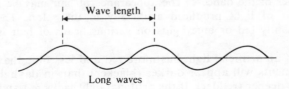

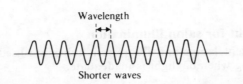

Fig. 8.3 Wavelength

The various colours of light also have different wavelengths, that of red being nearly twice as long as that of violet light. The short waves of violet light are refracted (bent) more than the longer waves of red light, causing the dispersion of white light on passing through a prism.

The electromagnetic waves may be classified according to wavelength as shown in Table 8.1.

Table 8.1   Electromagnetic waves

Type of energy	Wavelength	Use
Radio waves	long	Radio transmission
Television waves	↑	Television transmission
Micro-waves	decreasing	Cooking
Infra-red		Heat treatment
Visible light	↓	For sight. Photography
Ultra-violet		Sun-ray treatment
X-rays	very short	X-ray photography

The colour of objects

The molecules of pigment or dye contained in an object will absorb certain colours (wavelengths) of light and reflect others. The colours which are reflected to our eyes determine the colour we 'see'.

When we talk about the colour of an object we normally mean its colour in white light. A white pigment reflects all the colours in white light. A black pigment absorbs all the colours of white light and reflects none. A red pigment reflects only red light and absorbs all other colours. Similarly a blue pigment reflects blue light and absorbs the other colours.

The colour of an object may appear to change if it is viewed under different coloured lights. Thus objects seen under 'sodium' yellow street lights look quite different when viewed in daylight. As the spotlights at a discotheque vary in colour so too does the apparent colour of the hair and clothes of the dancers. The appearance of hair may be affected by the colour of light produced artificially in the salon. The effect of predominantly red or blue lights on various heads of hair is shown in Fig. 8.4.

Thus if an artificial light has more red and less blue than daylight, blue pigments will appear darker (blacker) than in daylight and red pigments deeper (redder). If the artificial light lacks red and has more blue than daylight, red pigments will appear darker and blue pigments deeper.

Sources of light for salon illumination

Tungsten filament lamps and fluorescent tubes are used to provide artificial lighting when daylight is inadequate.

Filament lamps

The glass bulb of an electric filament lamp (see Fig. 8.5) contains a coiled filament of tungsten wire. Tungsten metal has a high electrical resistance and a high melting point. When electricity flows through the filament it becomes white hot, the electrical energy being converted into light and heat. Filament lamps have a low efficiency since a large

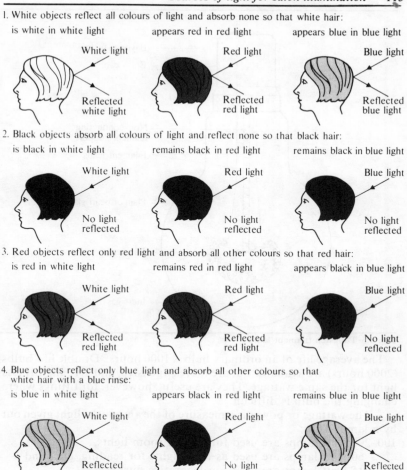

1. White objects reflect all colours of light and absorb none so that white hair:

    is white in white light   appears red in red light   appears blue in blue light

2. Black objects absorb all colours of light and reflect none so that black hair:

    is black in white light   remains black in red light   remains black in blue light

3. Red objects reflect only red light and absorb all other colours so that red hair:

    is red in white light   remains red in red light   appears black in blue light

4. Blue objects reflect only blue light and absorb all other colours so that white hair with a blue rinse:

    is blue in white light   appears black in red light   remains blue in blue light

Fig. 8.4 Effect of red and blue light on hair colour

proportion of the electricity is converted into heat. Bulbs of greater power than 60 watts should not be used in small enclosed fittings, as there is insufficient air movement in the restricted space to permit adequate cooling of the lamp.

The glass bulb enclosing the filament contains an inert gas such as argon or nitrogen. Air has to be removed as otherwise the hot filament would combine with oxygen and become less efficient. The filament may be a single coil or a coiled coil (see Fig. 8.6). The latter is more efficient as it emits the same amount of light as the single coil, for a lower consumption of electricity.

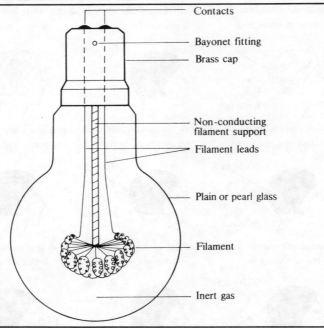

Contacts

Bayonet fitting

Brass cap

Non-conducting
filament support

Filament leads

Plain or pearl glass

Filament

Inert gas

Fig. 8.5 Tungsten filament lamp

The average life of an ordinary bulb is 1000 hours. 'Double life' bulbs (2000 hours) are available but are more expensive, and give slightly less light for the same wattage. They are useful, however, for fittings where changing the bulb is difficult.

The wattage or power is a measure of the amount of light given out by a lamp. Thus:

100–200 watt lamps are used for central room lights,

60 watt lamps are used as local lights for reading, etc., and

15 watt lamps are used for decorative purposes.

Most bulbs decrease in efficiency during their life. The shape of the lamp (bulb shaped or mushroom), however, has little effect on efficiency.

Filament lamps give a reddish-yellow light with less blue and green than daylight. This makes colour matching difficult. Blue and green shades appear darker and red shades brighter than in daylight.

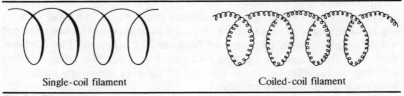

Single-coil filament

Coiled-coil filament

Fig. 8.6 Filaments.

Bulbs of various types are available:

1. Plain glass bulbs
The bright filament of this type of bulb may cause glare since the glass is transparent, and unless the bulb is shaded, eye strain may result. A plain glass bulb casts a sharp shadow.

2. Pearl bulbs
A pearl bulb is frosted on the inside so that the filament cannot be clearly seen. Glare is thus reduced, making it suitable for use where the lamp itself is visible.

3. Opal or silica coated bulbs
An opal bulb has an internal white coating which makes the whole bulb appear white, and the actual filament is not visible at all. There is a slight loss of light but the bulb appears uniformly bright, and this type of bulb is suitable when no lampshade is to be used.

4. Internally silvered bulbs
This type of bulb is used for spotlighting displays. The light is reflected by the silvered inner surface of the bulb, and the emergent beam is concentrated within a narrow angle (see Fig. 8.15).

Fluorescent tubes

In fluorescent tubes (see Fig. 8.7), an electric current is conducted through mercury vapour and this produces ultra-violet light. The inside of the

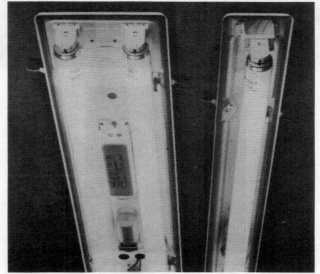

Fig. 8.7 Fluorescent tubes showing components

tube is coated with a fluorescent powder called a *phosphor* which converts the ultra-violet light into ordinary visible light. The colour of the light produced varies from a bluish white to a warm white according to the type of phosphor used. White fluorescent lighting has less red and

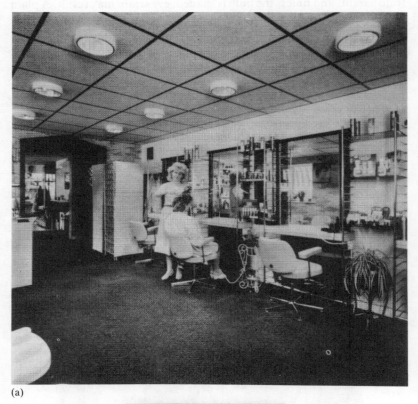

(a)

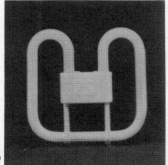

(b)

Fig. 8.8 (a) 'Cut Above' hairdressing salon, Penarth (Near Cardiff) using energy-saving Thorn EMI compact fluorescent 2D lamps.
(b) Thorn EMI's 16W 2D miniature fluorescent bulb.

yellow than daylight so makes blue and green pigments look brighter and red shades darker. 'Warm white' tubes give a light similar to daylight and are to be preferred for salon use. Fluorescent lighting of this type is thus more suitable for hair-colouring work than that from filament lamps. The tubes give a soft diffused light free from glare and casting very little shadow.

Straight fluorescent tubes are available in different lengths, the longer the tube the greater the wattage. Miniature fluorescent lamps (see Fig. 8.8), in which the tube is shaped into a more compact form, have been designed to replace filament lamps. They may be installed in special fittings or adapted for the lampholders previously only suitable for filament lamps.

Fluorescent tubes operate at a much lower temperature than filament lamps and convert less of the electrical energy into heat energy and therefore more into light energy. Thus fluorescent tubes are much more efficient than filament lamps. A fluorescent tube gives about three to four times as much light as a filament lamp of the same power. A miniature fluorescent lamp rated at 36 watts gives about the same amount of light as a 150 watt filament lamp. Fluorescent tubes are therefore cheaper to run. They also have five times the expected life of a filament lamp. This compensates for the greater cost of buying and possibly of fitting fluorescent tubes.

The cool running of fluorescent tubes also makes them particularly suitable for salon use, especially where artificial light is used continually throughout the day and where overheating of the salon may become a problem.

Lighting circuits

Cables for lighting circuits are usually embedded in the wall plaster, below floor boards or above ceilings (see Fig. 8.9). In modern installations they are sometimes enclosed in plastic trunking which runs on the surface

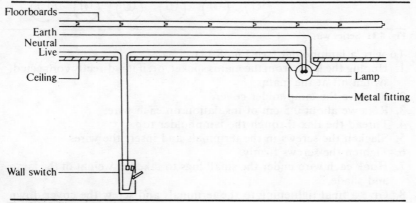

Fig. 8.9 Ceiling light with switch

of walls and ceilings so allowing easy access for later additions or modifications to the circuit. The cables are of suitable thickness to carry a
current of up to 5 A without overheating and the lighting circuit contains
a 5 A fuse in the consumer unit. Modern lighting circuits are provided
with an earth wire in order to safely earth metallic light fittings.

Room lamps are wired in parallel (see Fig. 8.10). With this arrangement
each lamp (or each group) is controlled separately by its own switch
which completes a closed circuit to the mains. The failure of one lamp
does not affect the use of the others.

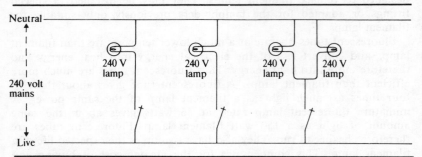

Fig. 8.10 Parallel wiring

Strings of coloured lamps used for the decoration of Christmas trees,
etc., are usually wired in series (see Fig. 8.11). If one lamp is removed or
damaged, all the lights go out as the circuit is broken.

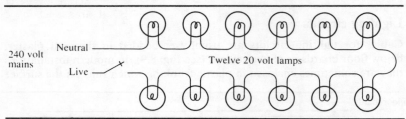

Fig. 8.11 Series wiring

To wire a lampholder (see Fig. 8.12).
1. Unplug the lamp from the mains socket, or, if it is directly connected,
   switch off at the mains.
2. Remove the lampholder cover.
3. Remove about 0·5 cm of insulation on each wire.
4. Thread the flex through the lampholder top.
5. Slacken the screws in the terminals and insert the wires.
6. Tighten the screws firmly.
7. Hook each wire under the small lugs to take the weight of the lamp
   and shade.
8. Give a final tightening to the terminals and screw the cover down
   firmly.

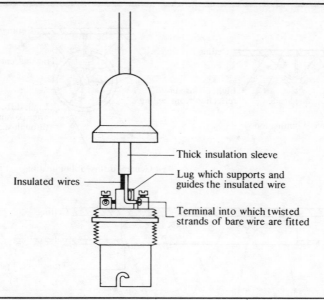

Thick insulation sleeve

Lug which supports and
guides the insulated wire

Insulated wires

Terminal into which twisted
strands of bare wire are fitted

Fig. 8.12 Re-wiring a lampholder

Light fittings

Light fittings may be designed either to give a uniform illumination over
the whole salon or to concentrate light on a small area such as a
particular working surface or a special display.

General purpose lighting for the whole salon may be achieved by several
methods:

1. *General diffused illumination* is produced when a filament lamp is
   enclosed in a translucent glass or plastic globe which diffuses the light
   as it passes through the shade (see Fig. 8.13), or when a fluorescent
   tube is enclosed in an opal plastic diffuser (see Fig. 8.14).

2. *Indirect illumination* results from a filament lamp concealed by an
   opaque fitting directing the light upwards to the ceiling. Reflection
   from the ceiling diffuses and distributes the light rays over the whole
   salon (see Fig. 8.13). The colour of the ceiling is particularly important
   in this case and should preferably be white so as to reflect the
   maximum amount of light.

3. *Luminous panels* concealing either filament lamps or fluorescent tubes
   behind sheets of translucent glass or plastic may be housed in a false
   ceiling (see Fig. 8.13). The whole ceiling acts as the source of
   illumination and a pleasantly diffused light is distributed over the room.

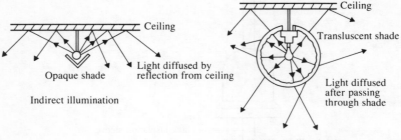

Ceiling

Opaque shade

Light diffused by reflection from ceiling

Indirect illumination

Ceiling

Transluscent shade

Light diffused after passing through shade

General diffused illumination

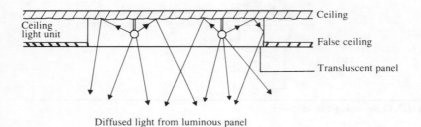

Ceiling

Ceiling light unit

False ceiling

Transluscent panel

Diffused light from luminous panel

Fig. 8.13 General purpose lighting

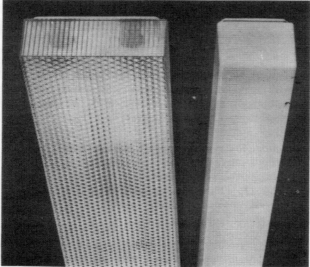

Fig. 8.14 *(Left)*   Prismatic controller used to direct light downwards
          (Right)   Opal diffuser used to scatter light in all directions

Localised lighting over small selected areas may be achieved by:

1. *Direct illumination* from a light fitting with a reflective shade which is arranged to direct about 90 per cent of the light downwards (see Fig. 8.15). *Spot light bulbs* also give direct illumination and when fitted to a track may be angled and positioned to illuminate special displays or pictures (see Fig. 8.15).
2. Fluorescent tubes may be fitted with clear *plastic prismatic controllers* containing a series of prisms which direct the light downwards in a chosen direction (see Fig. 8.14).

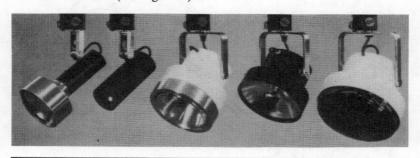

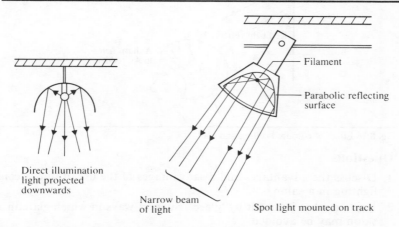

Filament

Parabolic reflecting surface

Direct illumination light projected downwards

Narrow beam of light

Spot light mounted on track

Fig. 8.15   *(Top)*   Spot-lights (photograph)
                 (Bottom)   Localised lighting

Effect of coloured ceiling and walls on salon lighting

The ceiling and walls of a salon should not be too deeply coloured as light reflected from them may affect the colour of objects in the room (see Fig. 8.16). The most suitable colour is white as there is little absorption of light, and no effect on colour.

Dark walls absorb light energy, and more light will have to be provided than if the walls have a light coloured finish with a good reflecting surface.

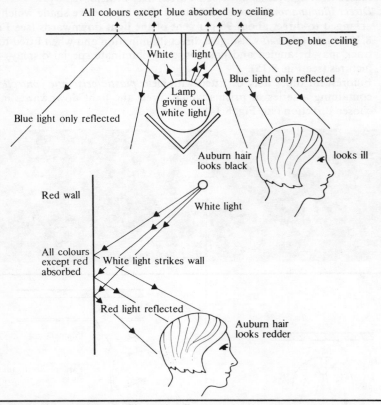

All colours except blue absorbed by ceiling

Deep blue ceiling

White   light

Blue light only reflected

Lamp giving out white light

Blue light only reflected

Auburn hair looks black

looks ill

Red wall

White light

All colours except red absorbed

White light strikes wall

Red light reflected

Auburn hair looks redder

Fig. 8.16 Effect of coloured ceiling and wall

Questions

1. Discuss the advantages and disadvantages of the use of fluorescent lighting in a salon.
2. Explain what is meant by 'glare'. Suggest ways in which glare in a salon may be avoided.
3. A head of auburn hair is observed:
   (a) in daylight;   (b) under a tungsten filament lamp;
   (c) under a 'white' fluorescent light;   (d) under a sodium street light.
   Explain any differences in colour which would be noticed.
4. Explain fully why it could be dangerous:
   (a) to drive nails into plaster walls;   (b) to change a filament bulb without switching off the current.
5. Explain what is meant by:
   (a) diffused lighting;   (b) a transparent substance;
   (c) a translucent substance;   (d) an opaque substance.

Chapter 9

The salon water supply

An adequate supply of both hot and cold water is required in a hairdressing salon. Besides the water used for various hairdressing processes including shampooing, water is required for washing gowns and towels and for general cleaning purposes. Cold water enters the salon by a service pipe from an underground mains supply, and the water must be heated as required. Although the mains water supply is sufficiently pure and safe for drinking and washing purposes, it is not chemically pure and often contains dissolved substances which may cause difficulty to the hairdresser. In addition to the mains supply, small quantities of chemically pure water are also required in the salon.

Cold water supplies

Water authorities take their supplies from reservoirs, natural lakes, deep wells, boreholes or from the upper reaches of rivers. Before

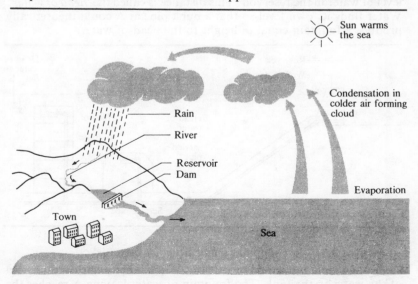

Fig. 9.1 The water cycle

collection the water has taken part in the natural water cycle (see Fig. 9.1).

Purification and treatment of the water is required before it enters the supply pipes.

1. The water is first stored in *sedimentation* tanks to allow large solid particles such as stones and soil to settle.
2. Smaller suspended particles are then removed by *filtration*. The water passes through filter beds containing graded layers of stones, gravel and sand.
3. *Aeration* of the water by bubbling air through it helps to kill germs and improves the taste of the water.
4. Mains water is tested frequently by the Health Authorities. If the bacterial level is unsatisfactory, *chlorination* of the water may be necessary to destroy germs. Water which has been contaminated by sewage may contain organisms causing diseases such as typhoid and dysentry, so is unsuitable for domestic use.
5. *Fluoridation* (addition of small quantities of fluorides to prevent tooth decay) is sometimes carried out if the natural occurring fluoride content of the water is low.

The main supply to a building

If the reservoir is above the level of the town, water will flow from the high level and be forced to the top of a building by water pressure (see Fig. 9.2). The pressure of water increases with depth. The pressure of water at A in Fig. 9.2 depends on the vertical distance between A and the level of water in the reservoir. This distance is called the '*head of water*'. Water finds its own level so that a burst pipe at A could theoretically produce a fountain equal in height to the head of water.

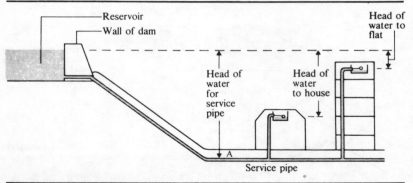

Fig. 9.2 Reservoir situated above town

Experiment 9.1   To show that water finds its own level.

Water flows from the nozzle A (see Fig. 9.3) if it is placed below the level of the water in the tank. The fountain of water leaving A reaches the same height as the level of the water in the tank. If the nozzle is at the same level or above the level of the water in the tank, the flow of water from the nozzle stops.

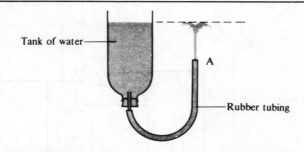

Fig. 9.3 Water finds its own level

If the reservoir is lower than the buildings requiring a supply (see Fig. 9.4), the water has first to be pumped into a water tower at a higher level, to provide the necessary head of water to force the water to the top of the tallest building.

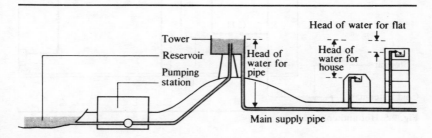

Fig. 9.4 Water supply where the reservoir is lower than the town

Water pressure from a reservoir or tower thus forces cold water into a tank placed high in a building (see Fig. 9.5), the level of the water being controlled by a ball valve. Water which has passed through the cold water tank is unsuitable for drinking because of possible contamination. Drinking water should be taken from taps directly connected to the mains. The rate of flow of water from taps supplied from the cold tank depends on the head of water between the tap and the level of water in the tank, the greater the head the faster the flow.

Stop-taps enable the supply to be cut off for repairs, for the replacement of tap washers, or if there are bursts in the pipes. One stop-tap is usually placed inside the building near the entry point of the supply, and another on the outlet of the cold water tank. Hairdressers should note the position of stop-taps so that these can be turned off quickly in an emergency, or if the building is to be left unoccupied for a time such as a holiday period.

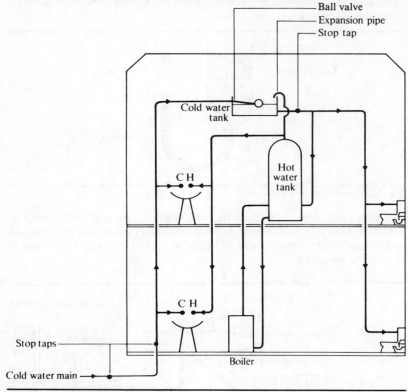

Fig. 9.5 Hot and cold water supplies

The hot water supply

There are various methods of heating water for salon use and it is essential to have a constantly available supply.

1. Hot water may be supplied from a *boiler* heated by gas, oil or solid fuel. Hot water rises by convection from the boiler to the top of a storage tank or cylinder from which it is drawn off to the basins (see Fig. 9.5). The boiler may form part of a central heating system, in which case hot water for the taps is heated indirectly through a heat exchanger in the hot water tank, and is kept separate from the water circulating through the radiators.

2. Water may be heated directly in the storage tank by an *immersion heater*. Heating often takes place at night using cheap off-peak electricity, but in salons with small tanks heating may be required during the day as well. The heating element is enclosed in a metal

sheath and may be inserted vertically from the top of the tank (see Fig. 9.6) or horizontally at either the top or bottom. Fitting an immersion heater at the top results in a quick accumulation of hot water at the top of the tank whilst the bottom remains cold. Hot water rises and since water is a poor conductor of heat no heat passes down the tank. A horizontal heater fitted at the bottom of the tank results in the gradual heating of the whole tank, since the water is constantly circulating by convection. Two-element heaters are available. These are fitted vertically and have a long element to heat the bulk of the water at night using off-peak electricity and a short element to keep the top part of the cylinder hot during the day. The temperature of the water in the hot tank is usually controlled at about 60°C by an adjustable thermostat.

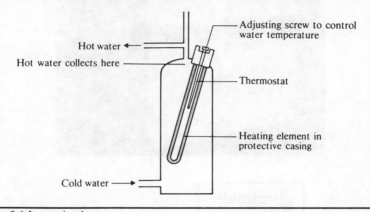

Fig. 9.6 Immersion heater

3. *Instantaneous water heaters* are connected to the cold water supply and the water is heated only as required. The temperature of the water is usually controlled by a thermostat. They are economical to run and are particularly suitable for the small salon. Both gas and electrically heated models are available. In gas heaters (see Fig. 9.7), a small pilot light constantly burning inside the heater lights the main jet as soon as the water begins to flow. Single point heaters may be fitted for each basin or a larger multipoint heater may supply several basins. The heaters are usually fitted with a balanced flue in an outside wall. In electrical installations each basin has its own heater. The water is heated rapidly as it passes over a high powered element. The temperature of the water is thermostatically regulated and depends on the rate of flow of the water and the loading of the appliance which may vary from 3 kW to 9 kW.

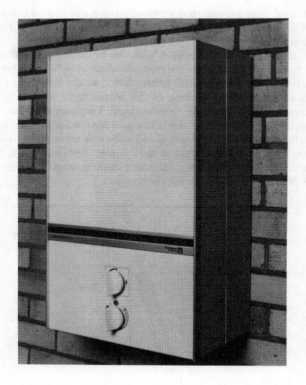

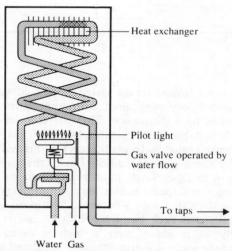

Heat exchanger

Pilot light

Gas valve operated by water flow

To taps ⟶

Water Gas

Fig. 9.7 Instantaneous water heater (gas)

Lagging

The insulation or lagging of hot water cylinders and pipes is essential if heat is not to be wasted. The lagging consists of a fitted jacket of any material which is a poor conductor of heat (see Fig. 9.8).

Cold water pipes on cold outer walls, and tanks in unheated roof space may also require lagging as a protection from frost damage. When water freezes it increases in volume by about one tenth. This expansion causes great pressure which may burst pipes or damage appliances. Glass-fibre, foam rubber or wool felting are suitable insulating materials.

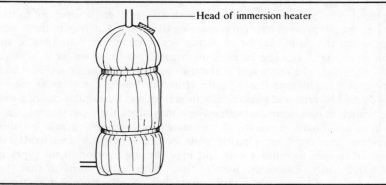

Fig. 9.7 Lagging jacket round hot water cylinder

Experiment 9.2   To compare the insulating properties of materials.

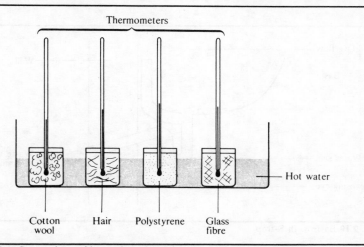

Fig. 9.9 Comparison of insulating properties

Set up the apparatus as shown in Fig. 9.9 using different insulating materials in each of the four identical copper vessels, which are placed in hot water. Note the temperature rise in each case over a period of 30 minutes. The container with the lowest temperature indicates the best insulator. Suitable materials are polystyrene, glass fibre, cotton wool and hair cuttings.

Shampoo basins

Shampoo basins are usually made of glazed stoneware or vitreous china which is easily kept clean using a non-abrasive cleaner. Cracked or chipped basins which will harbour germs and collect grease and dirt should be replaced. The basin should be fitted with a *filter* over the opening to the waste pipe, to prevent hair from entering the drain. The *trap* in the waste pipe under the basin may be an *S-trap* as shown in Fig. 9.10, or a *bottle trap* as in Fig. 9.11. The latter is often preferred in salons as it is more easily cleaned. The *water seal* in the trap prevents unpleasant odours and air-borne bacteria entering the salon from the drains. The *cleaning eye* or cap should be removed periodically to extract any accumulations of solid waste such as hair, soap and scum which may block the pipe. Hot washing soda solution may be poured down waste pipe to remove grease but this does not remove hair. Caustic soda solution (sodium hydroxide) is sometimes used to remove hair, but may cause corrosion of the pipes if used frequently. Basins are usually fitted with 'mixer' taps so that the temperature of the water is easily controlled. A mixer tap is sometimes controlled by a valve so that when the desired mix of hot and cold water has been achieved, the tap may be turned off and on again without altering the mix. Spray fittings are necessary to assist shampooing.

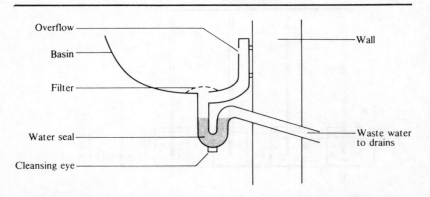

Fig. 9.10 Basin with S-trap

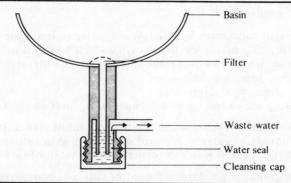

Fig. 9.11 Basin with bottle trap

Drains

The waste pipes from washbasins may join a pipe taking rain water from the roof, or may lead directly into a gully trap which is covered by a grating at ground level. The gully trap is fitted with a water seal and the trap should be cleaned regularly. Waste from the lavatories enters a separate pipe known as a soil pipe (see Fig. 9.12). In modern buildings the soil pipe is an internal pipe and the waste pipes from the washbasins may be connected to this pipe, thus avoiding exposed waste pipes outside the building.

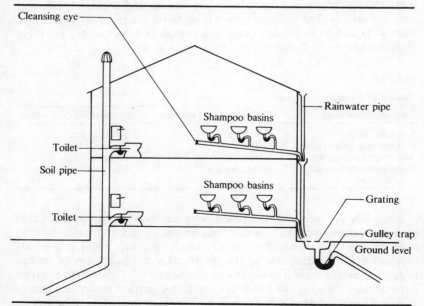

Fig. 9.12 Drains

Water as a solvent

Many different substances will dissolve in water so that water is rarely pure in nature. If a substance dissolves in water it is *soluble* in the water. The substance which dissolves is the *solute*, and the water is the *solvent*. Together they form a *solution*.

Solute + solvent = a solution

The following are examples of solutions with water as the solvent:

Citric acid crystals (solid) + water = citric acid solution (acid hair rinse)
Glycerol (liquid) + water = glycerol solution (a skin softener)
Formaldehyde (gas) + water = formalin (used in sterilising cabinets)

A solution containing a large amount of solute is *concentrated*. Tap water, which contains small quantities of dissolved salts, is a very *dilute* solution. If a solution contains as much solute as it can possibly hold it is a *saturated* solution. However, the amount of a solid dissolving in water may usually be increased if the temperature of the solution is raised. When the solute is a gas, it is driven out of solution by heat and so less gas dissolves at a higher temperature. This principle is applied in heating formalin to produce formaldehyde gas for the sterilisation of tools.

When acids, alkalis or salts dissolve in water some of their molecules split into two parts, one carrying a positive electrical charge and the other a negative electrical charge. These charged particles are called *ions*. Positively charged ions are termed *cations* and negatively charged ions are *anions*. The solutions containing them are *electrolytes* because they will conduct an electric current. Examples of electrolytes and their ions are shown in Table 9.1.

Table 9.1   Formation of ions.

Solution (electrolyte)	Positive ion (+) (cation)	Negative ion (−)(anion)
Sulphuric acid	Hydrogen ion	Sulphate ion
Sodium hydroxide (alkali)	Sodium ion	Hydroxyl ion
Sodium chloride (a salt)	Sodium ion	Chloride ion
Potassium oleate (a salt) (soft soap)	Potassium ion	Oleate ion

Acids always produce hydrogen ions as their cation and alkalis always produce hydroxyl ions as their anion. Pure water contains few ions, so does not conduct electricity easily, but tap water is a good conductor due to the ions of the dissolved salts. Solutions of many organic substances such as sugar and alcohol do not conduct an electric current since they do not ionise but contain complete molecules of the solute. Thus a solution may contain molecules or ions of the solute, and these are mixed evenly throughout the solution so forming a *homogeneous* mixture. Solutions are always transparent though they may be coloured. The particles in a solution are too small to be seen through a microscope.

If soap is dissolved in water, the particles present are larger than in a true solution. Such a solution is termed a *colloidal solution* and will remain cloudy even after filtering.

Dissolving is a *physical change*. The solute and solvent are just mixed together and are not chemically combined so no new substance has been formed. The solute is usually easily separated from the solvent. Solid solutes are left behind if the solvent is evaporated off by heating. Liquid and gaseous solutes may be separated by distillation.

Substances which will not dissolve in water are *insoluble* in water but may be soluble in a different solvent. Fats, for example, are insoluble in water but dissolve in trichloroethane, and this substance is used as a grease solvent in wig cleaning. Other solvents include alcohols (ethanol and isopropanol) used to dissolve resins in making hair lacquer, and amyl acetate used as a solvent for nail lacquer.

The hardness of water

Tap water often contains dissolved salts. The quantity and type of salts depends on the nature of the ground through which the rainwater passes on its way to the reservoir. For example, in limestone or chalky areas water may contain dissolved calcium or magnesium salts, but in areas of granite rock the water is relatively free from dissolved salts.

If the dissolved salts form an insoluble *scum* with soap before forming a lather, the water is said to be *hard*. Soft water contains few dissolved salts and forms an immediate lather with soap.

There are two types of hardness:

1.   Temporary hardness

This type of hardness is due to calcium bicarbonate or magnesium bicarbonate dissolved in water. These salts are formed when rainwater, made acid by dissolving carbon dioxide from the air, reacts with limestone or chalk as it runs through the ground.

Calcium carbonate   + carbon dioxide + water → calcium bicarbonate
(insoluble chalk   (soluble in water)
or limestone)   carbonic acid

Temporary hardness can be removed by boiling the water, when the above reaction is reversed and the calcium bicarbonate is decomposed or split up as follows:

Calcium bicarbonate → calcium carbonate + carbon dioxide + water
                              (insoluble scale)

Calcium carbonate is insoluble and is deposited as a *fur* or *scale*. This deposit of fur takes place in kettles and hot water pipes and boilers in hard water areas. Temporary hardness is often removed on a large scale by adding slaked lime to a town's water supply.

2. Permanent hardness

This type of hardness is caused by calcium sulphate or magnesium sulphate which is dissolved from the ground by rainwater. Permanent hardness cannot be removed by boiling, but is removed along with temporary hardness using chemical means.

The disadvantages of hard water

1. A *scum* or curd of calcium soap (lime soap) is formed when soap is used in hard water. This wastes soap, as no lather is formed until all the calcium and magnesium salts have reacted with the soap.

Calcium sulphate   + sodium stearate → sodium sulphate + calcium stearate
(permanent hardness)   (soap)   (soluble)   (insoluble scum)

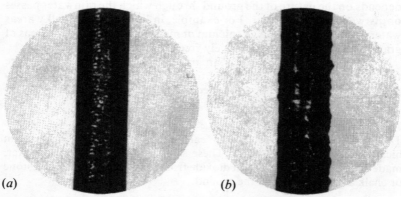

(a)   *(b)*

Fig. 9.13 (*a*) Hair washed in soft water. (*b*) Hair washed in hard water

No scum is formed if soapless detergents are used instead of soap. Soapless detergent shampoos are thus more satisfactory for use in hard water areas, and most modern shampoos are of this type. The use of soap shampoos in hard water results in a sticky deposit of scum on the hair and round the shampoo basin (see Fig. 9.13).

2. Temporary hardness produces *fur* or scale deposits in kettles, steamers, pipes and boilers. The circulation of water through central heating pipes may be impeded or stopped if the pipes become blocked. The scale is costly to remove and is damaging to equipment, besides making it less efficient.

The advantages of hard water

The disadvantages of hard water far exceed the slight advantage of a more pleasing taste, and a minor addition of calcium to the diet.

Methods of softening water

If water is hard, it usually contains salts causing both temporary and permanent hardness, though not necessarily in the same proportions. Both types of hardness can be removed by the following methods:

1. The ion exchange process (Permutit process) is the most satisfactory method for a salon, as the whole supply is softened by passing it through a water softener (see Fig. 9.14). This contains sodium ion-exchange resin which exchanges its sodium ions for the calcium ions in the hard water.

sodium resin   + calcium sulphate → calcium resin   + sodium sulphate
(water softener)   (in hard water)   (left in the   (dissolved in the
water softener)   softened water)

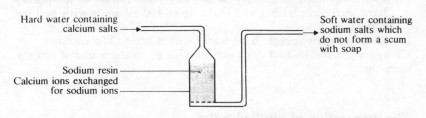

Fig. 9.14 A water softener

The water leaving the softener is not chemically pure as it contains dissolved sodium salts, but these do not form a scum with soap so the water is soft. The sodium resin in the water softener is gradually used up, and is replaced by calcium resin which will not soften water. However, the sodium resin may be reformed or regenerated by passing a strong solution of sodium chloride (common salt) through the water softener. This regeneration takes place automatically in modern water softeners.

calcium resin + sodium chloride → sodium resin + calcium chloride
                (salt)   (regenerated)   (in water run
                                                            to waste)

Water softeners used to contain a natural resin known as zeolite.

2. 'Calgon' or sodium hexametaphosphate is a sequestering agent (to sequester means to separate) and combines with calcium and magnesium ions, preventing the reaction between the soap and hard water, so that no scum is formed. Calgon is often added to shampoo and washing powders as a water softener. It is also used as a rinse after a soap shampoo to remove lime soap from the hair.

3. Other water softeners used in laundry work include ammonia, sodium carbonate (washing soda) and borax. Sodium carbonate is also used as a water softener in the form of bath salts. All these substances are alkaline and are not suitable for salon use.

Experiment 9.3   Comparison of hardness in water.
Fill a burette with standard soap solution. Place 25 ml of chemically pure water (distilled or de-ionised) in a conical flask. Add soap from the burette 0·5 ml at a time, shaking well after each addition. Note the amount of soap required to make a permanent lather, (a lather lasting for at least a minute). Repeat using each of the following:

(a) 25 ml of tap water;
(b) 25 ml of temporary hard water (prepared by bubbling carbon dioxide through lime water until the precipitate redissolves);
(c) 25 ml of permanently hard water (use 0·1% solution of calcium chloride);
(d) 25 ml of boiled temporary hard water (boil 100 ml of temporary hard water, cool, filter and make up to 100 ml again with purified water);
(e) 25 ml of permanently hard water with a little Calgon added.

Compare the results and draw conclusions as to the waste of soap in each case.

The preparation of purified water

Chemically pure water is required in the salon for use in the steamer and to dilute chemicals such as hydrogen peroxide. Purified water may be obtained from tap water by either distillation or de-ionisation. **Distillation** is a physical change involving the boiling of impure water to form steam, condensing the steam and collecting the pure water in a clean vessel. The apparatus used is shown in Fig. 9.15. Any impurities are left behind in the flask.

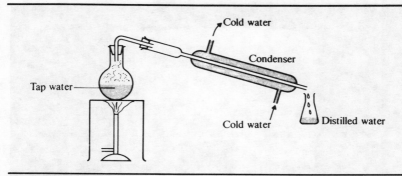

Fig. 9.15 Distillation

De-ionisation involves a chemical process similar to that of ion exchange water softening, but two columns of ion exchange resins are required (see Fig. 9.16a). De-ionised water is more often used than distilled water, as it is easier and cheaper to prepare. The portable de-ioniser shown in Fig. 9.16b contains a replaceable cartridge of resins and gives an immediate supply of de-ionised water when connected to a cold water tap.

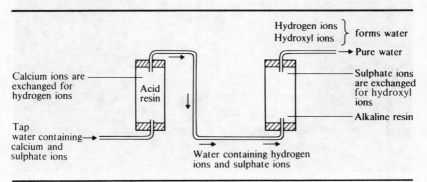

Fig. 9.16 (a) De-ionisation

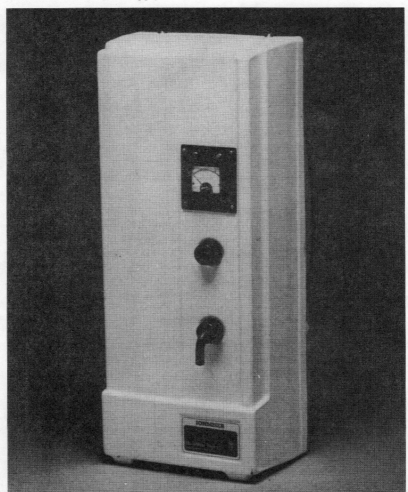

Fig. 9.16 (*b*) Portable de-ioniser

Questions

1. Classify the following processes into physical and chemical changes, giving the reason in each case:
    (a) making lacquer by dissolving plastic resin in alcohol;
    (b) shampooing hair;   (c) softening water by the ion exchange process;   (d) the formation of a scum when soap is used with hard water;   (e) the de-ionisation of water;   (f) the distillation of water.
2. What difficulties would you encounter if you opened a salon in a

hard water area? Describe how you would overcome the difficulties.

3. Explain why water pipes may burst in very cold weather and why the burst may not be noticed until the temperature rises. How would you deal with a burst pipe? What steps can be taken to avoid such an occurence?

4. Explain why:
   (a) tap water is a good conductor of electricity but pure water is not;   (b) water from a domestic cold tank is unsuitable for drinking;   (c) de-ionised water is used in the kettle of a steamer;   (d) the pressure of the water from a cold tap of a wash basin is often greater than the pressure of water from the hot tap.

5. Explain the difference between each of the following:
   (a) a physical and a chemical change;   (b) soft water and de-ionised water;   (c) a true solution and a colloidal solution.

Part 3
Hairdressing processes

Chapter 10

Shampooing the hair

The aim of shampooing is to cleanse the hair and scalp by the removal of dust, dirt, grease (mainly sebum), dead skin scales and various hair-dressing preparations such as lacquer or control creams. About twenty litres of water at a temperature of approximately 40°C are required during each shampoo so that the water is slightly above body temperature. Besides assisting in the removal of grease and dirt, massage of the scalp during shampooing increases the blood flow to the scalp so promoting healthy growth. Rinsing away the shampoo is important as flakes of shampoo dried in the hair may be mistaken for dandruff. Some shampoos are also hygroscopic and leave the hair sticky if not washed out completely. Conditioning rinses, added at the final rinse, help to ensure that the hair is in good condition after shampooing. The shampoo itself enables the cleansing process to take place effectively.

Shampoos
Shampoos may be divided into two groups:

1. Dry powder shampoos
These contain absorbent powders such as talc, starch, Fullers earth and French chalk, together with an alkali, usually borax or sodium carbonate (washing soda).
A typical formulation is:

Absorbent powder   80–85 per cent
Alkali   15–20 per cent
Perfume as required.

The mixture is sprinkled over the hair section by section in 2 cm partings, and is applied to the hair itself rather than to the scalp. The powder is left for 10–15 minutes to absorb the grease from the hair and is then brushed out systematically, the brush being wiped frequently on a clean towel to remove the dirt and powder. The method is not very satisfactory as it is difficult to remove all traces of powder, and this leaves the hair dull. Since brushing stimulates the activity of the sebaceous glands, hair tends to become greasy quickly after this type of shampoo.

2. *Detergents* (surfactants or surface active agents)

These include both *soaps* and *soapless* (non-soap) detergents. Strictly speaking a detergent is 'a substance which cleans' but it can be more accurately defined as a substance used with water to make things clean.

The soaps and most soapless detergents used as shampoos are known as *anionic detergents*, because the negatively charged anion of the detergent molecule is responsible for the cleansing action of the detergent.

Soft soap shampoos may contain potassium oleate. This separates into ions as follows:

Potassium oleate   →   potassium ion   +   oleate ion
                        (positively charged   (negatively charged
                        cation)   anion)

Soapless detergent shampoos may contain sodium lauryl sulphate which ionises as follows:

Sodium lauryl sulphate   →   sodium ion   +   lauryl sulphate ion
                              (positively   (negatively
                              charged cation)   charged anion)

In both cases the anion has a similar structure and consists of a negatively charged *hydrophilic* (water-loving) head, and a long *hydrophobic* (water-hating) tail (see Fig. 10.1).

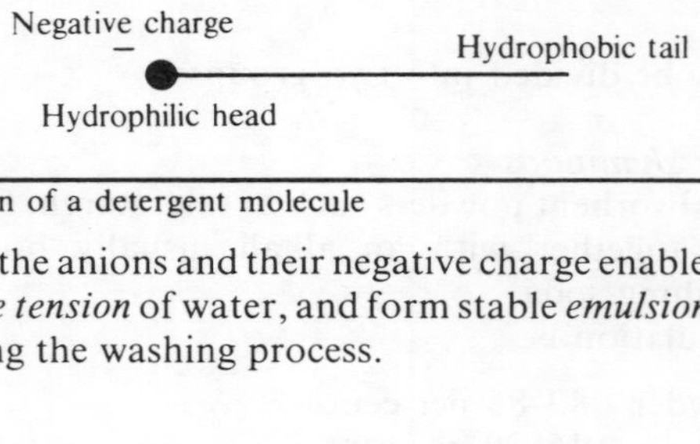

Negative charge

Hydrophobic tail

Hydrophilic head

Fig. 10.1 The anion of a detergent molecule

The structure of the anions and their negative charge enable the detergent to lower the *surface tension* of water, and form stable *emulsions* between water and grease during the washing process.

The surface tension of water

There are strong forces of attraction between the molecules in water. The forces at the centre of the liquid act in all directions (see Fig. 10.2) and balance each other. At the surface, however, the forces pulling the molecules inwards have practically no balancing forces acting outwards into the air. Thus the surface has an inward pull which creates surface tension, and this makes water act as though its surface has a 'skin'. It also causes contraction of the surface so that water has a tendency to form droplets and does not spread easily over surfaces.

When water is placed on a fabric it tends to remain in droplets and does not wet the fabric. For this reason water, by itself, is not a good

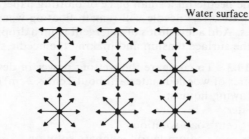

Water surface

The arrows show forces of attraction
between water molecules

Fig. 10.2 Surface tension

cleansing agent. If detergent is added to a drop of water on a fabric, the waterloving heads push in between the water molecules at the surface of the drop and the water-hating tails are forced out into the air. The detergent thus expands the surface, causing the droplets to collapse, spread and wet the fabric (see Fig. 10.3). The detergent is called a *wetting agent* or surface active agent.

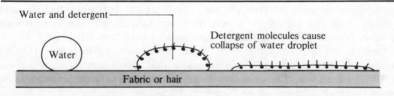

Water and detergent

Detergent molecules cause
collapse of water droplet

Water

Fabric or hair

Fig. 10.3 Lowering the surface tension

Experiment 10.1   To show the use of a detergent as a wetting agent. Place a few drops of water on a piece of woollen material using a dropping pipette. The water will form droplets on the surface of the fabric. Repeat using water containing a little shampoo. This will soak into the fabric immediately (see Fig. 10.4).

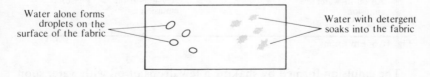

Water alone forms
droplets on the
surface of the fabric

Water with detergent
soaks into the fabric

Fig. 10.4 Wetting agents

Experiment 10.2   To demonstrate the surface tension 'skin' on water.
1. Completely fill a straight-sided vessel to the rim with water. Carefully slip small objects such as coins or buttons down the side of the vessel into the water which, held by the 'skin', rises above the surface of the vessel.

2. Place a fine needle on a small piece of blotting paper and float the paper on water. The needle will remain floating when the blotting paper sinks. Add a few drops of detergent from a dropper pipette so lowering the surface tension and making the needle sink.

Experiment 10.3   To compare the wetting power of detergents.
Float squares of woollen material (about 2 cm × 2 cm) on the surface of the following liquids:
(a) tap water
(b) 0·3 per cent soap solution
(c) 0·3 per cent sodium lauryl sulphate solution

Note in each case the time taken for the material to become wet and sink, so determining the best wetting agent. The wetting power of various types of shampoo can also be tested by this method.

Emulsions

An emulsion consists of minute droplets of one liquid suspended in another liquid. The two liquids must be insoluble in each other. All emulsions consist of two phases, the droplets forming the *disperse phase,* and the liquid in which they are suspended, the *continuous phase.* Most common emulsions consist of mixtures of oil and water. Droplets of oil suspended in water form an *oil-in-water* (O/W) emulsion, and droplets of water suspended in oil form a *water-in-oil* (W/O) emulsion. The droplets in an emulsion are large enough to be seen through a microscope (see Fig. 10.5).

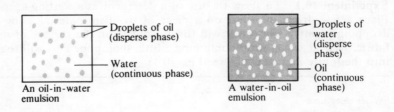

Fig. 10.5 Emulsions

The emulsion formed by shaking a few drops of oil with water soon separates into two layers. To prevent this a third substance, an *emulsifying agent*, must be added so making the emulsion permanent. Detergents, lanolin, cetrimide (a cationic detergent) and synthetic emulsifying waxes such as Lanette wax (a mixture of cetyl and stearyl alcohols) act as emulsifying agents. The molecules of the emulsifying agent lower the surface tension and form a bridge between the two liquids by surrounding the droplets of the disperse phase (see Fig. 10.6).

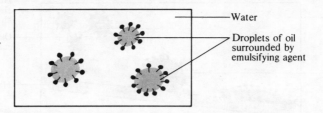

Fig. 10.6 Emulsion showing position of emulsifying agent

Many cosmetic creams and lotions, such as conditioning creams and barrier cream, are emulsions. Detergent acts as the emulsifying agent for the emulsion of water and grease formed during shampooing.

Experiment 10.4   To illustrate the difference between a solution and an emulsion.

Solution. Place a few grains of salt on a microscope slide and add a drop of water. Cover, and watch the salt dissolve whilst under the microscope. The salt disappears from view because the salt dissolves into particles which are too small to be seen through a microscope.

Emulsion. Make an emulsion by shaking a few drops of olive oil with water containing a little detergent. Place a few drops of emulsion on a microscope slide, cover and examine through the microscope. The drops of oil are plainly visible, showing that the particles in an emulsion are much larger than in a solution.

Experiment 10.5   Detections of emulsions.

Spread drops of various hairdressing preparations very thinly on separate microscope slides. Cover and examine each under a microscope to decide which are emulsions. Test perm lotions, conditioning creams, shampoos and bleaches.

How detergents clean hair

Detergent shampoos work in the following way:

1. By acting as wetting agents

The detergent lowers the surface tension of the water so spreading the water over the surface of the hair and bringing it into closer contact with the hair.

2. By acting as an emulsifying agent

The anions of the shampoo molecules have negatively charged waterloving heads, and long tails which are attracted to grease. During shampooing, the tails of the anions enter the grease whilst the heads stay in the surrounding water (see Fig. 10.7*a*). The negative charges on the

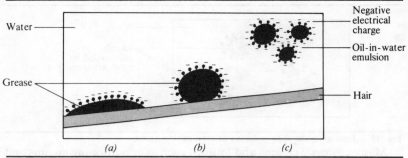

Fig. 10.7 Detergent action

heads of the ions repel each other, causing the grease to roll up (see Fig. 10.7*b*), become dislodged from the hair and form an oil-in-water emulsion (see Fig. 10.7*c*). Hot water and rubbing also help to dislodge the grease from the hair. Solid particles of dirt (particulate dirt) are removed along with the grease.

3. By acting as suspending agents for the grease

The droplets of grease in the emulsion repel each other due to the negative charge on the detergent ions which surround the grease. Thus the droplets are prevented from joining together to form larger globules which could be re-deposited on the hair. The grease remains suspended in the water until it is rinsed away.

The qualities of a good shampoo

A good surfactant shampoo should have the following qualities:
1. It should spread easily over the surface of the hair.
2. A rich creamy lather should be produced. Although some detergents will clean efficiently without one, a lather is important in washing hair and skin, since it provides a concentrated solution of detergent which is easily moved over the surface of the skin or scalp. A lather also acts as a visible guide to the amount of detergent required.
3. It must be a good wetting agent, yet must not make the hair so wet that it is difficult to dry out. During shampooing, hair may soak up to 30 per cent of its own weight in water. Drying must reduce that amount to the normal 10 per cent of moisture in hair.
4. Whilst being a good emulsifying agent, it should not de-grease the hair and scalp excessively as this may lead to dermatitis and dry unmanageable hair.
5. The shampoo should be a good suspending agent so that grease is not re-deposited on the hair shafts.
6. It should be easily rinsed out of the hair.
7. The hair should be left manageable and lustrous when dry.
8. The shampoo should not irritate the eyes or skin by being either too acid or too alkaline.

Comparison of soap and soapless detergents

It is difficult to distinguish between soap and soapless shampoos except by testing them chemically. They may look alike and act similarly during shampooing if the water is soft, but they are different chemical substances with different properties and are made by different processes.

Experiment 10.6   To compare the method of preparation of soap and soapless detergents.

Both soap and soapless detergents may be prepared from vegetable oils (usually castor oil, coconut oil and olive oil).

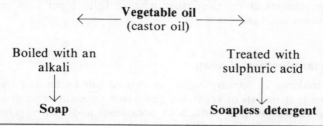

The preparation of a soap	The preparation of a soapless detergent
Dissolve 2 g of sodium hydroxide in 10 ml of water in a small beaker. Warm the solution with 2 ml of castor oil and stir until boiling. (*Care* – sodium hydroxide burns the skin.) Boil gently for 3–4 minutes. Add 10 ml of de-ionised water and 6 spatula measures of common salt. Boil again for 2–3 minutes. Allow to cool. Filter off the solid and wash it on a filter paper with de-ionised water and allow to dry. Shake a small quantity of the solid with water in a test-tube. A lather is produced from the soap.	Using a teat pipette add 2 ml of concentrated sulphuric acid to 1 ml of castor oil in a boiling tube and stir with a glass rod (*Care* – sulphuric acid burns the skin.) Heat is produced and the contents become brown and thick. Transfer the contents to a boiling tube half filled with water. Stir to remove the excess acid. Pour off the water, carefully retaining the solid. Wash twice more with water. Shake a small quantity of solid with water in a test-tube. A lather is produced from the soapless detergent.

Comparison of the properties of soap and soapless detergent

Soap shampoo	Soapless shampoo
Alkaline so roughens the cuticle. pH = 8–9	Neutral so leaves the hair smoother than soap shampoo. pH = 7
Forms a scum with hard water	No scum with hard water
Decomposed by acids	Unaffected by acids, so used in acid shampoos
Insoluble in salt solution	Salt is used to thicken these shampoos
May become rancid	Unlikely to become rancid
Rarely cause dermatitis	Often cause dermatitis
Better suspending power	Better wetting agents. Better removal of grease. May de-grease the hair too much

Experiment 10.7 Comparison of properties of soap and soapless shampoos.

Make up a soap solution by dissolving one spatula measure of soap flakes in 50 ml of warm de-ionised water. Make a similar solution using sodium lauryl sulphate (soapless detergent). Using equal quantities of each in separate test-tubes, carry out the following tests:
1. Test for acidity or alkalinity using litmus paper.
2. Find the pH value of each using pH paper.
3. Add a little acetic acid to each and note any collapse of foam.
4. Test with a little hard water and note any formation of scum.
5. Note any salting out when salt is added.
6. Note the effect on the lather when a little 1 per cent cetrimide solution is added.

The manufacture of soap

Soap making, or *saponification*, is carried out by boiling animal fat (beef or mutton fat) or vegetable oil (castor, coconut or palm oil), with strong alkalis such as sodium or potassium hydroxides. The manufacturer adjusts the type of fat or oil and the type of alkali according to the soap required.

Hard soaps are used in toilet soap and soap powders and are made by boiling animal fats with sodium hydroxide. They consist mainly of sodium stearate and sodium palmitate which are the sodium salts of stearic and palmatic acids.

Glyceryl stearate + sodium hydroxide→sodium stearate + glycerol
    (fat)   (alkali)   (hard soap)

Glycerol (glycerine) is formed as a by-product. The soap and glycerol are separated by 'salting out' with brine. Soap is insoluble in common salt solution and so floats to the top. The glycerol is refined and used in skin lotions, hand creams and as a plasticiser (a softener of plastic) in lacquers.

Soft soaps which are used in shampoos are made by boiling vegetable oils with potassium hydroxide.

Vegetable oils + potassium hydroxide→potassium oleate + glycerol
                (alkali)   (soft soap)

In this case there is no salting-out process and the glycerol is left in the soap. Soft soaps and shaving soaps are sometimes made by the neutralisation of stearic acid or oleic acid by potassium hydroxide.

Oleic acid   + potassium hydroxide→potassium oleate +   water
Acid   + alkali   = a salt   + water

The formulation of shampoo from soft soap

Soft soap shampoos are made by the dilution of soft soap with varying proportions of water and industrial methylated spirit. Spirit shampoos are useful as *lacquer-removing* shampoos.

Example: Green soft soap 45 g.
Industrial methylated spirit 5 ml.
Water 50 ml.
Perfume as required.

The manufacture of soapless detergent shampoos

1. Sulphonated oils

These oils, such as sulphonated castor oil, are used in conditioning shampoos. They act as an oil and a detergent at the same time and are easily rinsed off the hair. Their manufacture is represented by the following equation:

Castor oil + sulphuric acid ⟶ Sulphonated castor oil
                                      (also called Turkey Red oil)

A typical oil shampoo contains:
Sulphonated castor oil 15 per cent
Sulphonated olive oil 15 per cent
Water 70 per cent.

2. Sulphated lauryl alcohols

These form the largest group of shampoos. Lauryl alcohol is obtained from coconut oil, and is then treated with sulphuric acid to form lauryl hydrogen sulphate. Neutralisation by various alkalis gives a range of neutral surfactants used as shampoos.

Lauryl alcohol + sulphuric acid = lauryl hydrogen sulphate

The formation of various detergents and their properties are shown in Table 10.1. Some modern shampoos are based on sodium lauryl ether

Table 10.1   Preparation of shampoos

	Alkali	Surfactant	Properties of surfactant
Lauryl + hydrogen sulphate	sodium hydroxide	→ sodium lauryl sulphate	A white paste used in cream shampoos. Not suitable for clear shampoos as it is not very soluble in cold water.
Lauryl + hydrogen sulphate	ammonium hydroxide	→ ammonium lauryl sulphate	A thick amber liquid.
Lauryl + hydrogen sulphate	triethanolamine	→ triethanol-amine lauryl sulphate (T.L.S.)	A thin colourless liquid. Very mild. Used in clear liquid shampoos.
Lauryl + hydrogen sulphate	monoethanol-amine	→ monoethanol-amine lauryl sulphate	Thicker than T.L.S., so easier to apply. Mild.

sulphate, which is milder than sodium lauryl sulphate and more soluble in cold water, so is suitable for clear as well as cream shampoos.

3. Coconut imidazoline

Coconut imidazoline is prepared from coconut oil or synthetically from petroleum products. Very mild shampoos designed as baby shampoos and for use on delicate or damaged hair are formulated with up to 20 per cent coconut imidazoline. Sebum is not produced until a child is four or five years old so these shampoos often contain a low percentage of detergent. They also have a very low eye irritancy.

The formulation of soapless shampoos

Soapless shampoos are available in several forms:

Clear liquid shampoos

These may contain triethanolamine lauryl sulphate, ammonium lauryl sulphate, or sodium lauryl ether sulphate.

Example:

Triethanolamine lauryl sulphate 20 per cent
Coconut monoethanolamide 2 per cent (improves lather)
Water 78 per cent
Perfume and colour traces

Liquid cream shampoos

These are similar to clear liquid shampoos but are thickened by the addition of soap which makes the shampoo opaque.

Solid cream shampoos contain:

Sodium lauryl sulphate	25 per cent
Soap	5 per gent
Water	70 per cent

Gel shampoos

These contain 20–25 per cent of triethanolamine lauryl sulphate thickened with methyl cellulose to a semi-solid, jelly-like consistency.

Powder shampoos

These are not very popular as they have to be dissolved in warm water before use. They contain spray dried sodium lauryl sulphate.

Aerosol shampoos

Sodium lauryl sulphate and triethanolamine lauryl sulphate may be dispensed as an aerosol foam. These detergents, however, are corrosive to metals so the aerosol container is often made of glass with a plastic outer cover. Sodium lauryl sarcosinate is less corrosive and is therefore more frequently used. The shampoo foams as it leaves the container due to the propellent gas passing through the detergent solution. Aerosols are considered more fully at the end of this chapter.

Additions to soapless shampoos

Perfume and colour are usually added to shampoos to increase their appeal. Soapless shampoos may also be modified in various ways by the addition of the following ingredients:

1. Lanolin, egg, beer and citric acid are added as *conditioners* to make the hair more manageable.
2. Sodium alginate, soap, or common salt are used as *thickeners*.
3. Sodium hexametaphosphate is added as a *water softener*.
4. Camomile may be used as a *brightener* for blonde hair.
5. Henna and walnut juice are added to *colour* shampoos.
6. Hexachlorophane, bithionol, coal tar and resorcinol are *antiseptics* used in medicated shampoos.
7. Formalin is a *preservative* and prevents bacterial growth in shampoos.
8. Selenium sulphide and zinc pyrithione are *keratolytics* (keratin splitters), which are added to antidandruff shampoos to remove scales of keratin.
9. Protein hydrolysates consist of mixtures of individual amino acids and short polypeptide chains of amino acids which cling to hair electrostatically so are said to be *substantive* to hair. They act as *conditioners*, making the hair smoother and improving lustre.
10. Lauryl diethanolamide is added as a *foam stabiliser*.

The perfuming of shampoos

Shampoos and other hairdressing preparations are perfumed by the addition of sweet-smelling *essential oils*, which are obtained from various parts of plants as shown in Table 10.2. The oils are *volatile*, so evaporate readily at room temperature, the molecules of oil stimulating the nerve endings in the nose to give rise to the sense of smell (see Fig. 10.8). Other vegetable oils such as castor oil and olive oil are not volatile and are referred to as 'fixed oils'.

Table 10.2   Essential oils

Part of plant	Name of oil
Leaf	Oil of bay, thyme, petitgrain (orange leaves)
Flowers	Oil or attar of roses, jasmin, lavender, neroli (orange flowers) and ylang ylang
Peel of fruit	Oil of lemon, orange and bergamot
Grasses	Citronella
Bark	Cinammon

Essential oils are extracted from plant material in several ways:

1. By *steam distillation*.
2. By *extraction with a solvent* such as petrol or petroleum ether.
3. By *pressing* the peel of citrus fruits.
4. By *enfleurage* or absorption of the oil from flower petals by contact with lard, so forming a pomade.

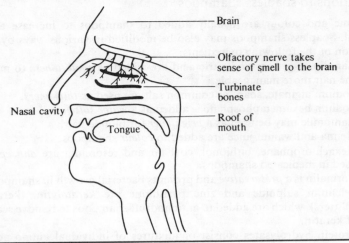

Fig. 10.8 Section through the face

In the formulation of perfumes, various essential oils may be blended together. Certain *animal secretions*, which are not in themselves sweet smelling, are added to the oils to equalise the rates of evaporation of the oils so that the perfume has the same scent over a long period. The animal secretions include ambergris obtained from the intestines of sperm whales, castor from beavers, musk from the musk deer of Tibet, and civet from the civet cat of Ethiopia. To make skin perfumes, the oils and animal secretions are dissolved in industrial methylated spirit.

Some essential oils such as oil of cade, oil of bay and oil of rosemary have antiseptic properties and are used in medicated shampoos and hair tonics. They are not as effective as modern synthetic antiseptics.

Conditioning rinses

Conditioning rinses are applied to the hair at the last rinse after shampooing.

Acid rinses will remove the scum of lime soap and neutralise traces of alkali left on the hair after use of a soap shampoo. They close the cuticle scales making the hair smoother and easier to comb. Vinegar rinse (acetic acid) contains 50 ml of vinegar per litre of warm water and is often used on dark hair. Lemon rinse (citric acid) contains 10 g of citric acid crystals dissolved in a litre of warm water and is suitable for blonde hair.

Beer and egg rinses give 'body' to the hair, by slightly stiffening the hair on drying. They aid setting and add lustre to the hair.

Cream rinses contain quaternary ammonium compounds such as cetrimide (cetyl tri-methyl ammonium bromide). These substances are also known as *cationic detergents* since the active part of the detergent is the positively charged cation. They cannot be used at the same time as anionic detergents such as soap and the lauryl sulphates (where the active part of the molecule is negatively charged), since the opposite charges cause destruction of the detergent properties. It is therefore essential to wash out all traces of shampoo before using the rinse. Cetrimide is an antiseptic as well as a detergent and may be used alone as an anti-dandruff shampoo. A film of cetrimide is left clinging electrostatically to the hair even after rinsing. Hair normally has an excess of negatively charged acid groups, which attract the positively charged cations of cetrimide making cetrimide *substantive* to hair. Cetrimide rinses make hair easier to comb and prevent fly-away hair due to static electricity. Care must be taken in using cetrimide as it is damaging to the eyes.

Shaving preparations for men

In men, the terminal hair of the beard area is usually fairly coarse. The follicles themselves are often large and may have two distinct openings, one for the hair shaft and the other for the sebaceous gland. Although the short hairs of a cut beard seem stiff and bristle-like, the beard when grown is usually quite soft. To obtain a comfortable shave this bristle-like hair must first be softened by water. A shaving preparation of soap or cream must also be applied to lubricate the skin, so enabling the razor to slip easily over the skin surface to avoid skin damage. The soap or cream also holds the hairs erect so that they can be easily cut. The razor itself must be very sharp.

Several types of shaving preparations are available:

1. *Shaving soaps*
   Shaving soaps may be in the form of a solid stick or a soft cream contained in a tube. They must lather freely with water and be non-irritant, so must contain no free alkali. The soap is usually superfatted by the addition of vegetable oils to reduce alkalinity to a pH of 8. Mixtures of hard and soft soaps are used. Shaving sticks contain one part of hard soap to two parts of soft soap. Tube soaps contain one part of hard soap to five parts of soft soap. Lanolin may be added as an emollient (skin softener) and menthol as an astringent to cool the skin.

2. *Brushless shaving creams*
   Brushless creams are oil-in-water emulsions containing 15–20 per cent of mineral oils and a small quantity of triethanolamine soap to give a pH of 8. Traces of silicone oils may be added to improve the spreading properties of the cream. The emulsion should be thick enough not to drip. It should rinse away easily and not leave the skin sticky. Since brushless creams do not soften hair easily the beard area should be washed with soap and water immediately before the cream is applied.

3. Aerosol foams

Oil-in-water emulsions similar to, though not as thick as, brushless shaving creams may be dispensed as a foam from an aerosol container. The preparation consists of 92 per cent cream and 8 per cent aerosol propellant. On leaving the can the propellant vaporises and expands, producing bubbles as it passes through the watery detergent phase of the emulsion.

After-shave lotions

After-shave lotions are designed to cool the skin, soothe any discomfort due to slight skin damage and apply a mildly antiseptic film to the shaving area. They consist of alcohol and other astringents such as witch hazel or menthol, together with antiseptics and perfume. The evaporation of the alcohol requires latent heat which is taken from the skin.

A typical lotion contains:

Industrial methylated spirit (astringent)	60 ml
Water	40 ml
Glycerol (skin emollient)	3 ml
Menthol (astringent)	0·05 g
Cetrimide (antiseptic)	0·1 g

Aerosols

A wide variety of hairdressing preparations including shampoos, shaving creams, setting lotions and lacquers are now produced as aerosols. In addition to the main ingredients of the product, the aerosol can also contains *a propellant* which forces the product out of the can when the nozzle is pressed (see Fig. 10.9).

The propellant is a highly volatile liquid (often a halogenated hydrocarbon such as chlorofluoromethane) and so the liquid easily turns to vapour at room temperature. The vapour always fills the space above the product in the can and creates a pressure on the surface of the liquid. When the can is opened to the atmosphere by depressing the nozzle, the pressure of the vapour inside the can pushes the liquid contents of the can out since its pressure is much greater than the opposing pressure of the outside air. The vapour pressure inside the can stays the same whether the can is full or nearly empty, so that the spray comes out at the same speed throughout the life of the aerosol. The fineness and type of spray is determined by the size and shape of the opening in the nozzle. In the case of shampoos, shaving creams and setting lotions which contain detergent, the product foams as it leaves the can. Some of the liquid propellant also leaves the can when the nozzle is pressed. This liquid vaporises and expands, so bubbling through the detergent creating a foam as it passes out into the air. In aerosol setting lotions, the foam is designed to break down quickly on the hair.

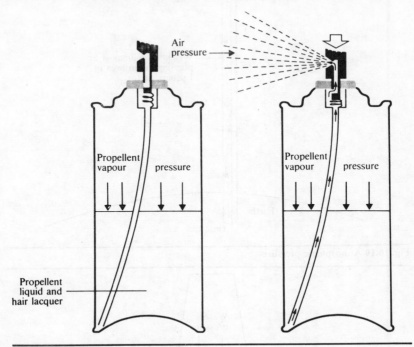

Fig. 10.9 The working of an aerosol can

Atmospheric pressure

Atmospheric pressure is due to the weight exerted on the earth by the layer of air surrounding the earth (see Fig. 10.10). Pressure is measured as the weight acting on unit area. The instrument used to measure atmospheric pressure is the *barometer*.

Pressure is expressed in newtons per square metre (N/m^2). A force of 10 newtons is approximately equivalent to the force exerted by a 1 kilogram weight.

The size of the atmospheric pressure is about $100\,000$ N/m^2.

This is equivalent to $10\,000$ kilogram spread uniformly over a square metre, or 1 kilogram on a square centimetre.

The pressure of the vapour inside an aerosol can is about three times as great as atmospheric pressure.

Experiment 10.8   To demonstrate atmospheric pressure.

1. Fill a glass tumbler completely with water and place a sheet of paper over it, making sure that there are no air bubbles under the paper. Turn the tumbler over carefully (over the sink!). The water does not fall out, because the air pressure is greater than the pressure of the water in the tumbler (see Fig. 10.11).

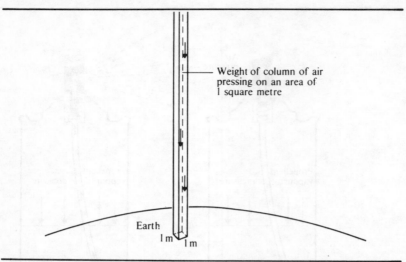

Fig. 10.10 Atmospheric pressure

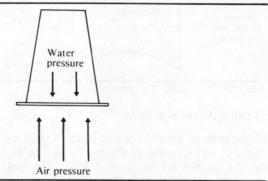

Fig. 10.11 To demonstrate air pressure

2. Obtain a tin with a screw cap – an old large-size motor oil tin is suitable. Remove the cap and heat a small quantity of water in the tin until it boils and fills the space above with steam, most of the air having been driven out. Quickly screw on the cap and remove the heat at the same time. Allow the tin to cool. Some of the steam condenses, creating a partial vacuum in the tin. The air pressure outside therefore crushes the sides of the tin, which are not strong enough to withstand the pressure (see Fig. 10.12).

Precautions in the use of aerosols

1. Store the cans in a cool place. Heat increases the pressure in the can by making more liquid turn to vapour, so that the can may explode if overheated.

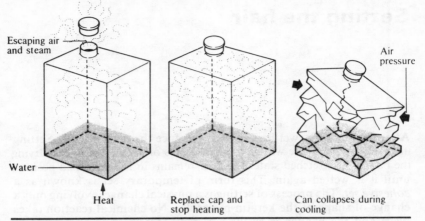

Escaping air and steam — **Air pressure**

Water —

↑
Heat | **Replace cap and stop heating** | **Can collapses during cooling**

Fig. 10.12 To demonstrate air pressure

2. Never place 'empty' aerosol cans on a fire. They will still contain vapour and may explode.
3. Do not puncture the can even if you think it is empty. It may still contain some vapour and liquid, which would spray out with considerable force.
4. If the nozzle becomes blocked, do not try to pierce it.
5. Read the manufacturer's instructions first before use, and always obey them.

Questions

1. Explain why regular washing of the hair and scalp is necessary. List the substances which may be removed during the process.
2. Why is shampoo a more effective cleanser than water alone?
3. Using the knowledge that pressure $= \dfrac{\text{Weight or force,}}{\text{area}}$ explain why
   (a) floor surfaces can be damaged when people wear shoes with heels having a very small area;
   (b) scissors are more efficient when sharp;
   (c) low heels on shoes are less tiring for the wearer than are high heels.
4. Explain why soapless detergent shampoos are more often used than soap shampoos. What are the disadvantages of soapless shampoos?
5. Explain why:
   (a) dry powder shampoos are less efficient than soapless detergent shampoos;
   (b) a good lather is important in a shampoo;
   (c) a soap shampoo must be rinsed from the hair before applying a cetrimide rinse.
6. What is meant by (a) lanolin; (b) an astringent; (c) an emollient; (d) an emulsifying agent?

Chapter 11

Setting the hair

After shampooing, wet hair is set to produce the desired style. Setting involves stretching the wet hair round rollers or with a brush and drying the hair in its stretched state. The hair remains in this stretched position until it is wetted again. This form of temporary set is known as a *cohesive set*. The process of setting is a physical change involving only a change of shape of the keratin molecules. No chemical reaction takes place and the change is easily reversed. This may be contrasted to permanent waving which gives a permanent set and requires chemical changes to the structure of keratin. It is, however, the chemical structure of keratin which makes it possible to carry out a cohesive set.

The chemical structure of keratin

Since keratin is a protein it is built up from *amino acids*, and there are eighteen different amino acids in hair. The amino acid molecules are chemically united by *peptide linkages* to form long chains called *polypeptide chains*.

The formation of a polypeptide chain is represented below:

amino acid —— amino acid —— amino acid —— amino acid
  molecule   molecule   molecule   molecule

peptide linkages or bonds

In the cortex, the polypeptide chains lie along the length of the hair in a spiral or coiled spring formation known as an α-*helix*. The coils are held together by weak *hydrogen bonds* which form between a hydrogen atom in one amino acid, and an oxygen atom in the amino acid lying immediately above or below it in the next turn of the spiral. Hydrogen bonds also occur between two adjacent polypeptide chains (see Fig. 11.1).

Other cross linkages also occur between adjacent polypeptide chains, resulting in a network or ladder-like structure.

Salt linkages or bonds are due to electrostatic attraction between the acid part of an amino acid in one polypeptide chain, and the amino (or basic) part of an amino acid in the adjacent chain. These bonds are weak and are easily destroyed either by acids or alkalis.

Cystine linkages are cross linkages in the amino acid cystine. Each molecule of cystine forms part of two adjacent polypeptide chains with the cystine linkage making a bridge between the chains. The cystine linkages each contain two sulphur atoms which are held by a *disulphide bond*. This type of bond is stronger than the salt and hydrogen bonds but may be broken by the chemical action which takes place during perming.

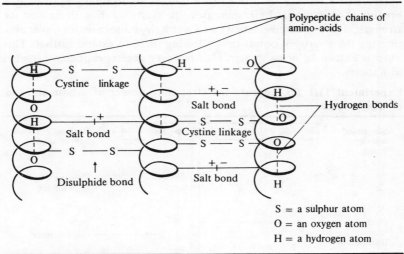

S = a sulphur atom
O = an oxygen atom
H = a hydrogen atom

Fig. 11.1 The structure of keratin

The elasticity of hair

Hair is elastic due to the coiled spring structure of the keratin in the cortex, which allows it to stretch and to spring back to its original length when released. The scales of the cuticle slide over each other to allow the hair to stretch. The amount of stretching is limited by the hydrogen bonds which hold the coils of the spring together, for although they are weak they are very numerous.

Keratin in unstretched hair is known as α-*keratin* (alpha-keratin). If the hair is stretched, some of the hydrogen bonds are broken and the spiral structure straightens out to form β-*keratin* (beta-keratin). When the stretching force is removed α-keratin is re-formed. The change on stretching is called the α-β transformation of keratin and is reversible. (Alpha is the first letter of the Greek alphabet and beta the second.)

$$\text{α-keratin} \xrightarrow[\text{released}]{\text{extended}} \text{β-keratin}$$

α-keratin   → β-keratin
(unstretched hair)   (stretched hair)

If hair is stretched with sufficient force, a point is reached when the hair will no longer return to its original length when the force is removed. The hair has then reached its *elastic limit*. When stretched beyond this limit a sudden extension of the hair may take place due to the breaking of a large number of hydrogen bonds. If the stretching force is again increased the hair eventually breaks, due to the breaking of the polypeptide chains.

Dry hair stretches by a third to a half of its original length before breaking. Wetting a hair increases its elasticity but decreases its strength. The increased elasticity of a wet hair is due to water molecules entering the hydrogen bonds thus allowing them to extend further. This water is known as *'bound'* water. Hair has even greater elasticity if treated with steam.

Experiment 11.1 To measure the stretching power of a hair and the breaking force.

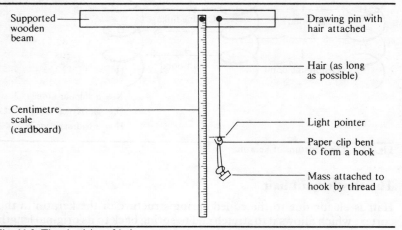

Fig. 11.2 The elasticity of hair

1. Set up the apparatus as shown in Fig. 11.2, using as long a hair as possible. Attach a loop of cotton to several 5 g and 10 g masses so that they may be suspended easily from the paper clip hook.
2. Measure the length of the hair, after fixing the paper clip which will help to keep the hair straight.
3. Add 5 g to the clip and leave for several minutes to allow stretching to take place.
4. Continue to increase the stretching force by 5 g or 10 g at a time, supporting the weight with the hand at each addition to prevent a sudden increase in tension. Note the length of the hair after each addition, always allowing time for stretching.
5. Note the number of grams required to break the hair.
6. Repeat the experiment several times using different hairs.
7. Work out the results as shown in Table 11.1.

Table 11.1 Typical results

Original length (in cm)	Length on breaking (in cm)	Stretch (in cm)	$\dfrac{\text{Stretch}}{\text{Original length}}$	No. of grams causing hair to break
18	24	6	$\dfrac{6}{18} = \dfrac{1}{3}$	90
20	26	6	$\dfrac{6}{20} = \dfrac{1}{3}$ approx.	80
27	40	13	$\dfrac{13}{27} = \dfrac{1}{2}$ approx.	100

The cohesive set

The setting of hair depends on its ability to stretch, so that hair which is over-processed or very dry does not take a good set due to lack of elasticity. The stretching of dry hair is limited by the hydrogen bonds, and to obtain a greater extension setting is carried out on wet hair. Water molecules enter the hydrogen bonds between the coils so allowing the hair to stretch further. Stretching is achieved by winding the hair tightly on rollers, or by the movement of the brush in blow-drying. The hair is dried in this stretched state so remains in the β-keratin condition. During drying, the water held in the hydrogen bonds is evaporated off. Since the hair is still under tension, the bonds re-form at a different point along the polypeptide chain (see Figure 11.3). The hair is thus set in its stretched position and does not spring back to its original length when the rollers are removed. The set is not destroyed until the hair is wet again.

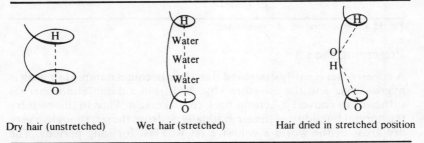

Dry hair (unstretched)   Wet hair (stretched)   Hair dried in stretched position

Fig. 11.3 Cohesive set

Experiment 11.2. To demonstrate a cohesive set.

Make a bundle of about 12 hairs of equal length (the longer the better, but not less than 20 cm) and knot them together at each end. Suspend the hair as shown in Fig. 11.4 and measure the length between the knots. Stretch the hairs by adding a mass of 200 g. With a 50 ml pipette, run hot water containing a little shampoo down the hairs until they are thoroughly wet. Allow time for the hairs to stretch and then note the new length. Remove the stretching force and dry the hair with a hand dryer. Note that the hair returns to its original length. Stretch the hair again, wetting it as before. Now dry the hair with the 200 g still in position, removing it only when the hair is perfectly dry. Note that the hair now remains at its stretched length. The hair has been set. Wet it with cold water and the hair will return to its original length.

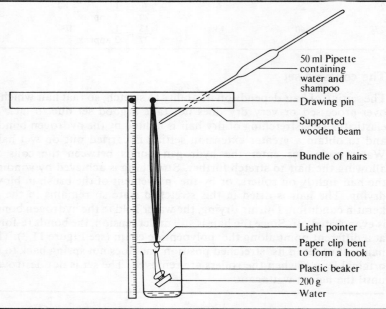

50 ml Pipette containing water and shampoo

Drawing pin

Supported wooden beam

Bundle of hairs

Light pointer

Paper clip bent to form a hook

Plastic beaker

200 g

Water

Fig. 11.4 Demonstration of cohesive set

Preserving the set

A cohesive set is easily destroyed if the hair becomes damp. Hair itself is hygroscopic, and the moisture absorbed from a damp atmosphere is sufficient to convert β-keratin back to α-keratin. Thus in this country the normal humidity of the air gradually destroys the set, though in very dry areas of the world a cohesive set will last for long periods. The absorption of moisture is reduced by the natural surface coating of sebum and by applying conditioning creams, setting lotions and lacquer.

It is important that the air in the salon itself should not be excessively humid, or the set may be destroyed before the client leaves the salon. A wall hygrometer should be used to indicate the level of humidity in a salon, and humidity should be controlled by good ventilation.

Experiment 11.3 To demonstrate the action of sebum and lacquer. Obtain six cubes of sugar. Cover two cubes on all sides with cold cream to produce a similar effect to sebum. Cover two more with a coating of hair lacquer. Leave the remaining two cubes untreated. Place the cubes in a shallow layer of coloured water as shown in Fig. 11.5. Note that the water rises in the untreated cubes, but is prevented from rising by the cold cream and lacquer.

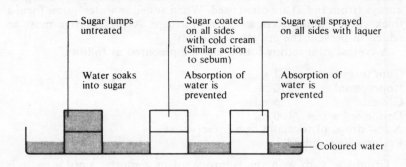

Fig. 11.5 Action of sebum and lacquer

Temporary heat setting

A temporary heat set may be obtained by moulding the dry hair into the desired shape by heated irons (Marcel waving), crimping irons, heated rollers or heated styling brushes. The hair is both heated and stretched at the same time, then allowed to cool under tension. New hydrogen bonds are formed in a different position in the polypeptide chains, a greater number of bonds being involved than in a cohesive set. The new bonds are completely destroyed by hot water but only slightly by cold water. Hot water is therefore required to break the set.

Hot pressing, using a heated pressing comb, is a form of heat setting used to straighten over-curly negroid-type hair. Pressing oil, containing petroleum jelly or a thick emulsion of silicone oils, is applied to the hair before combing. This lubricating oil reduces friction damage to the hair and also acts as a heat transfer agent which facilitates the conduction of heat from the comb to the hair. The heated comb stretches the hair as it is straightened against the comb surface. Frequent hot pressing may lead to bald patches (traction alopecia) due to excessive dragging on the hair during combing. Setting the hair on large heated rollers is a less damaging alternative.

Setting lotions

Setting lotions prevent the hair from drying out too quickly during setting, and help to preserve the life of the set by preventing moisture from entering the hair shaft.

There are two main types of setting lotions:

1. Gum setting lotion

Gums are carbohydrates which are obtained from certain trees when the bark is damaged. The gum forms an exudation from the wound, and is picked off the trees by hand. Gum tragacanth (from Turkey) and gum karaya (from India) are often used. When added to water, gums form a thick sticky solution known as *a mucilage*. A preservative must be added to prevent the growth of moulds.

A typical gum setting lotion may be prepared as follows:

Gum tragacanth   1 g
Isopropanol   10 ml
Glycerol   5 ml
De-ionised water   100 ml
A few drops of formalin as a preservative
Perfume as required

Grind the gum with the isopropanol in a mortar until a paste is formed. Add the water and stir vigorously. Add glycerol, preservative and perfume.

2. Plastic setting lotion

Most modern setting lotions contain plastic resins such as dimethyl-hydantoin formaldehyde resin (DMHF) or polyvinyl pyrrolidone (PVP), dissolved in a mixture of alcohol and water. The plastic resin is left as a film on the hair when the water and alcohol have evaporated.

A typical formula is:

Polyvinyl pyrrolidone   2 g
Industrial methylated spirit   20 ml
De-ionised water   80 ml
Glycerol   4 ml
Perfume as required

Dissolve the resin in the alcohol (industrial methylated spirit) and water. Add the glycerol and perfume. The glycerol acts as a *plasticiser* to soften the plastic film left on the hair after drying.

Plastic setting lotions may be *coloured*, giving the hair a temporary colour which will wash out at the first shampoo.

A typical formula for a brown coloured setting lotion is:

Co-polymer polyvinyl pyrrolidone/polyvinyl acetate   2 g
1 per cent solution Sunset Yellow   10 ml
1 per cent solution Erythrocine (red)   2·5 ml
1 per cent solution Sulphan Blue   0·75 ml
De-ionised water   40 ml
95 per cent ethanol   45 ml
Perfume as required

These setting lotions may also be formulated with detergent solution for use in aerosols. The lotion emerges from the aerosol can as a foam which is designed to be unstable and to break down quickly on the hair.

Plastic setting lotions intended for use during blow drying often contain silicone oils which lessen friction and produce a heat-resistant film which helps to prevent hair damage by accidental contact with the blow dryer nozzle. Protein hydrolysates may be added as conditioners.

Questions

1. Explain what happens to the molecules:
   (a) of water and alcohol when a setting lotion dries on the hair;
   (b) when ice melts;
   (c) of a piece of metal whilst it is being heated.
2. Explain what is meant by each of the following:
   (a) elasticity;   (b) the elastic limit;   (c) a solution;
   (d) humidity;   (e) a plasticiser.
3. A setting lotion is made by dissolving 1 g of plastic resin in a mixture of 10 ml of alcohol and 40 ml of water. What quantities of each ingredient would be required to make a litre of setting lotion?
4. With what instrument would you measure the following?
   (a) 25 ml of water accurately;   (b) 0·75 ml of dye;   (c) 80 ml of water;   (d) the humidity of the air;   (e) the air temperature of the salon.
5. What steps can a hairdresser take to ensure that a cohesive set will be long lasting?

Chapter 12

Drying and dressing the hair

The final drying of hair may be carried out using a salon hood-dryer, a hand blow-dryer or an infra-red dryer, the water being removed by evaporation in each case. A hood-type dryer is used after roller setting and the dried hair is then dressed out into the desired style. Blow drying involves first blotting the hair with a towel to absorb sufficient water to prevent dripping, then simultaneously setting and drying the hair to its completed style, using a brush and blow dryer. Infra-red dryers are useful in cases where movement of the hair during drying is undesirable.

Towel drying

Towel drying is usually carried out immediately after shampooing to absorb surplus water, but still leaving the hair sufficiently wet to allow the hair to stretch easily during setting. A towel consists of loosely woven cotton threads between which are narrow air spaces. Water is drawn up into these air spaces by a surface tension effect known as *capillary rise*. Water is also absorbed into the fibres of the towel itself.

Experiment 12.1   To demonstrate capillary rise.

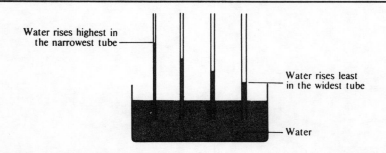

Water rises highest in the narrowest tube

Water rises least in the widest tube

Water

Fig. 12.1 Rise of water in capillary tubing

Support several glass capillary tubes of different bore in a dish of coloured water as shown in Fig. 12.1, and note that the water rises highest in the narrowest tube and least in the widest tube. This effect of capillary rise is due to a force of attraction between the water molecules and the molecules of the glass tube, and is a surface tension effect.

The structure and working of a hair dryer

Both hood and hand-held blow dryers consist basically of an electric motor which turns a fan, so blowing cold air over an electrically heated element (see Fig. 12.2). The motor converts electrical energy into mechanical energy to turn the fan. The heating element is made of nichrome wire which has a high resistance and so converts electrical energy into heat energy. In hood-type dryers the heating element and

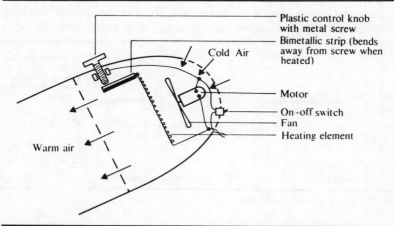

Fig. 12.2 Hair dryer

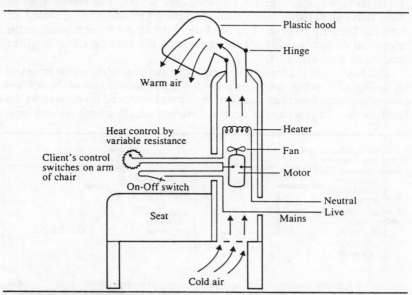

Fig. 12.3 Hair dryer — seating unit

motor are often enclosed in the hood itself, but increased efficiency is obtained by using a more powerful heater and motor placed behind the seating arrangement for the dryer, the hot air then being ducted to the hood. The client's control switches are then situated in the arm of the chair (see Fig. 12.3).

The working temperature of the dryer can be controlled in the following ways:

1. Thermostatic control

A thermostat is a device for keeping a piece of equipment working automatically at a constant temperature, and often consists of a

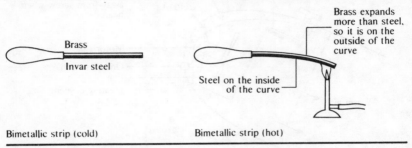

Fig. 12.4 The working of a bimetallic strip

bimetallic strip. This is a strip of two metals such as brass and invar steel, bonded firmly together all along their length. The metals must be such that one expands much more than the other whilst being heated, so causing the strip to bend. The bending of the strip causes a break in the electrical circuit, cutting off the current to the heating element of the appliance (see Fig. 12.4).

In a hair dryer the bimetallic strip touches the control screw (marked A in Fig. 12.5) when the dryer is cold. The insulated knob of the control screw is situated on the outside of the dryer hood, and is adjusted by the hairdresser. Thus when the dryer is switched on, the circuit is completed

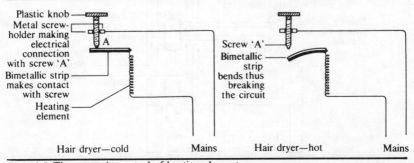

Fig. 12.5 Thermostatic control of heating element

and the heating element becomes hot. The heat developed in the dryer hood then causes the bimetallic strip to bend away from the screw. This breaks the circuit and so stops the flow of current through the heater. As the dryer cools, the strip straightens and makes contact again, so allowing the current to flow and heating to take place. The bimetallic strip thus operates as an automatic switch.

The temperature at which the bimetallic strip switches off the current is determined by the position of the control knob as shown in Fig. 12.6.

Since the motor is connected in parallel with the heating element, the working of the thermostat does not affect the fan, which continues to rotate as long as the dryer is switched on at the mains. If the fan becomes faulty a thermal cut-out mechanism will prevent the overheating of the appliance.

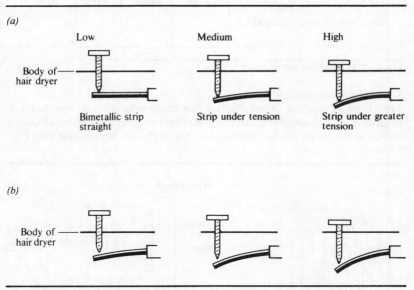

Fig. 12.6 Adjustments of the thermostat (*a*) Current flowing (*b*) No current

2. *Three-heat control switch*

The client often controls the temperature of the dryer by using a three-way switch held in the hand. This switch has three positions (low, medium and high) as well as an 'off' position, and controls the heating element in the dryer hood. The element may be considered to be in two sections, A and B, and the arrangement of the elements corresponding to the position of the switch is as shown in Fig. 12.7.

	Resistance	Current	Power (Watts)	Temperature
Low A B (Both elements used in series)	High	Low	Low	Low
Medium A or B (One element only is used)	Less	Higher	Higher	Higher
High A B (Two elements used in parallel)	Still lower	Much higher	Much higher	Much higher

Fig. 12.7 Three-heat control switch

3. *Variable control switch*
This type of switch is similar to the three-way switch but has ten positions each controlling different sections of a resistance, so allowing different amounts of current to flow through the heater coil (see Fig. 12.8).

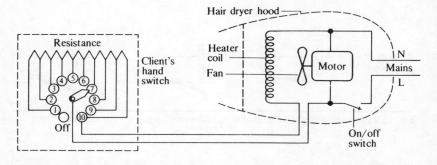

Fig. 12.8 A client's hand control

Drying by use of a hair dryer

A hair dryer is designed to provide suitable conditions for the rapid evaporation of moisture from the hair. During evaporation water changes state from a liquid to a vapour. Latent heat is required for this change, and if no external heat is supplied heat is taken from the client's head, so producing a cooling effect. A hair dryer supplies this heat, giving energy to the water molecules, making them move faster and enabling them to escape from the surface of the water into the air. The greater the heat supplied, the faster the molecules move and the quicker the evaporation of moisture. Evaporation takes place at any temperature but occurs more rapidly as the temperature rises.

If the surrounding air inside the dryer hood is saturated with moisture, it can hold no more and evaporation cannot take place. The hair dryer fan constantly moves moist air from around the wet head so allowing water to evaporate more quickly. If the cooler air entering the dryer from the salon is also humid, this will slow the drying process. The effect may be avoided by good salon ventilation.

Evaporation also takes place faster when a large surface of hair is exposed to the air. Thus hair is dried more quickly by blow drying when the hair is being constantly spread out by the brush, than if it is wound on rollers and dried under a hood dryer.

Experiment 12.2   To demonstrate the conditions affecting evaporation.
1. To show the effect of high temperature and movement of air.
    (a) Using a pipette, run 5 ml of water on to a large metal plate. Dry, with a hand hair dryer at 'cold', recording the time for complete evaporation.
    (b) Repeat with the same quantity of water, in the same place, using the hair dryer at 'hot'.
    (c) Repeat, leaving the water to evaporate in the natural state of the air without using the dryer, so that no forced air movement nor heat is involved.
    (d) Compare the times taken for evaporation in each of the three different conditions.
2. To show the effect of surface area.
    Pour 100 ml of water into each of the following vessels (see Fig. 12.9) and leave for about a week.
    (a) a 100 ml measuring cylinder;
    (b) a 250 ml beaker;
    (c) a trough about 20 cm diameter. Measure in each case, the volume of water remaining after a week.

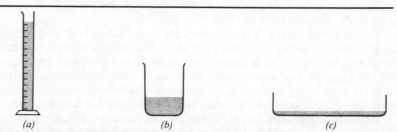

(a)   *(b)*   *(c)*

Fig. 12.9 To show the effect of surface area on evaporation

3. To show the effect of the humidity of the surrounding air.
   Pour 100 ml of water into each of two similar beakers. Cover one of
   the beakers with a bell jar (see Fig. 12.10). Keep the two close together
   to remain undisturbed for a week. Note the difference in water loss.

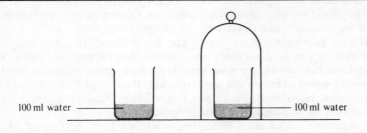

100 ml water —————   ————— 100 ml water

Fig. 12.10 To show the effect of humidity on evaporation

Infra-red dryers

The introduction of precision cutting and the styling of hair during
drying has led to the development of infra-red hair dryers (see Fig.
12.11). Styling can thus be undertaken without the hair being blown out
of place. Hand models contain a 275 watt infra-red lamp. Stand dryers
have three to five lamps, each with their own switch, mounted on
flexible metal arms which may be positioned in any desired direction.
The lamps are more comfortable for the client than traditional dryers
and noise is eliminated. Drying takes place by evaporation.

Dressing and controlling the hair

After drying the hair, rollers are removed and the hair is dressed out by
brushing and combing it into the required style. Since at this stage the
hair is very dry and has had the sebum removed by shampooing,
frictional electricity may be produced making the hair difficult to
manage (see Chapter 7). This effect is reduced by the use of a cetrimide
rinse after shampooing. The application of control creams or
brilliantine before dressing out also reduces the amount of static
electricity produced on the hair.

Control creams and brilliantines replace the natural oils and so help
to preserve the set by preventing the entry of atmospheric moisture into
the hair shaft. Since oil increases the reflection of light from the surface
of the hair, control creams add lustre to the hair. Although control
creams have been less popular since the introduction of cetrimide rinses,
aerosol-sprayed control dressings are often used after dressing out.

Both control creams and brilliantines may contain vegetable oils such
as castor oil or almond oil, but more often are based on mineral oils

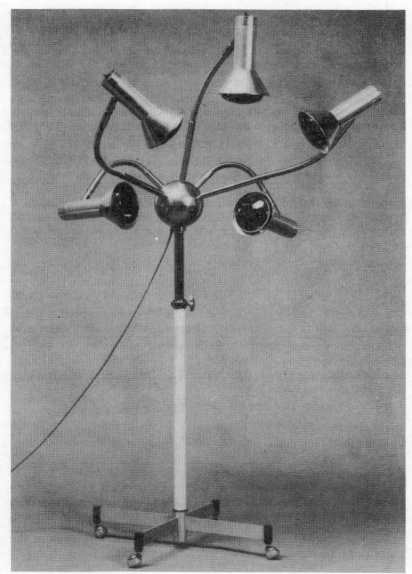

Fig. 12.11 Infra-red dryer

which are obtained from the ground as *petroleum products*. These substances are mainly *hydrocarbons* containing only the elements hydrogen and carbon. The distillation of petroleum produces the following main groups of substances:

(a) gases such as North Sea Gas, which are used for heating purposes;

(b) petrol;

(c) naphtha (white spirit) — used as a solvent for cleaning wigs;

(d) liquid paraffin and paraffin oil ⎱ used in control

(e) soft paraffin and petroleum jelly (Vaseline) ⎬ creams and

(f) paraffin wax ⎰ brilliantines

(g) pitch

Liquid brilliantines consist of mineral oils such as deodourised thin paraffin oil or sometimes castor oil (a vegetable oil), along with a suitable perfume.

A typical brilliantine contains

castor oil	15 ml
light paraffin oil	85 ml
perfume as required	

For spraying after dressing out the oil is dissolved in alcohol, and 100 ml of a typical brilliantine would contain:

castor oil	15 ml
industrial methylated spirit	85 ml
perfume as required	

Solid brilliantine is a mixture of liquid paraffin and soft paraffin with the addition of paraffin wax.

It may be prepared from the following formula:

liquid paraffin	20 ml
soft paraffin	70 g
paraffin wax	5 g
carnauba wax	5 g
perfume as required.	

Heat the ingredients gently after shredding the wax and stir until homogeneous. Add the perfume after cooling to about 40°C.

Control creams are usually oil-in-water emulsions with soap as the emulsifying agent.

A control cream may be prepared using the following ingredients:

Group A		Group B	
stearic acid	3·5 g	triethanolamine	1·5 ml
spermaceti wax	3 g	water	47 ml
liquid paraffin	45 g		

Heat both groups A and B separately to 70°C. Pour A into B, stir until cool and then add the perfume.

Triethanolamine (an organic base) and stearic acid react together to form triethanolamine stearate (a soap) which is the emulsifying agent. (Refer back to the chapter on shampoos if you need a reminder about the meaning of emulsions and emulsifying agents.)

Some control creams, particularly those used in men's hairdressing, are water-in-oil emulsions which become liquid when rubbed between the hands before application to the hair. The water phase allows the setting of the hair before it evaporates, leaving an oily film on the hair to impart gloss.

Clear micro-gel preparations are available in which mineral or vegetable oils are dispersed in water as sub-microscopic particles. These gels feel less greasy than ordinary oil-in-water emulsion control creams.

Greaseless gels contain propylene glycol as the fixative and are formulated with alcohol and water thickened with methyl cellulose to give a gel consistency.

Lacquers

After the dressing of the hair is completed, the style may be kept in place by a coating of lacquer. This also keeps moisture out of the hair and so protects the set. Lacquers have a similar composition to setting lotions, but contain less water as they are sprayed on to the dry hair and must not damage the set. They may be applied either by a puffer or an aerosol spray. Lacquers consist mainly of a solvent which evaporates quickly (usually industrial methylated spirit or isopropanol) and a solute which acts as the film former (usually shellac or plastic resin). When the solvent evaporates, a film of resin is left on the hair. A lacquer shield should be used to protect the client's eyes and prevent inhalation of fumes. Lacquer solvents are flammable and should not be sprayed near naked flames.

Shellac-based lacquer

Shellac is a natural resin obtained from India or Malaysia. It is produced by female lac insects which surround their bodies with the resin as they cling to the bark of certain trees during the production of young. The resin is collected from the trees by hand, purified and sold in the form of orange-coloured flakes, or is bleached and powdered.

Shellac has a strong holding power but tends to leave the hair stiff. It is insoluble in water but soluble in alcohol and in borax solution. Consequently it is necessary to use a lacquer-removing shampoo containing spirit or borax to dissolve it from the hair. Lanolin, a substance obtained from sheep's wool and similar in composition to sebum, is often added to shellac-based lacquers as a plasticiser, to make the lacquer more pliable.

Shellac   +   Alcohol   =   Hair lacquer
(solute)   (solvent)   (a solution)

A shellac-based lacquer may be prepared as follows:

bleached shellac	8 g
triethanolamine	2 ml
industrial methylated spirit	70 ml
water	10 ml

Dissolve the shellac in the industrial methylated spirit and then add the water mixed with the triethanolamine.

Plastic resin lacquers

These modern lacquers are usually based on co-polymer polyvinyl pyrrolidone/polyvinyl acetate or on dimethylhydantoin formaldehyde resin as the film former. The usual solvent is some form of alcohol (industrial spirit or ethanol). A small amount of glycerol or isopropyl myristate is added as a plasticiser to keep the plastic soft and make it less likely to flake on the hair. Silicone oils are often added to give a good spread over the hair.

Plastic resin	+	Alcohol	=	Hair lacquer
(solute)		(solvent)		(a solution)

A typical formula for a plastic resin lacquer is as follows:

co-polymer PVP/PVA 60/40	4 g
Isopropyl myristate	1 ml
silicone fluid	0·1 ml
absolute ethanol	80 ml
perfume as required	

This type of lacquer is designed for package in aerosol cans, and so contains no water. Indeed, water must be avoided in aerosols as it reacts with some propellants forming acids which may corrode the tin after a period of time.

Questions

1. Explain what is meant by
   (a) capillary rise;   (b) a bimetallic strip;   (c) a hydrocarbon;
   (d) an aerosol propellant.
2. Which electrical appliances in a salon depend for their operation on
   (a) an electric motor;   (b) a heating element?
   Which salon appliances are fitted with a thermostat?
3. List the electrical equipment used in a salon, stating the power in watts of each. In each case calculate the cost of running the appliance for 1 hour. (Assume that one unit of electricity costs 6p.)
4. What are the main causes of humidity in a salon?
   Describe the effect of high humidity on:
   (a) the people in the salon;   (b) the setting and drying of hair.
5. Give examples of each of the following:
   (a) a mineral oil;   (b) a vegetable oil;   (c) an essential oil.
   Explain their uses in hairdressing.

Chapter 13

Bleaching

Natural hair colour depends largely on the type and amount of pigment contained in the cortex of the hair. The pigments include *melanin*, which may be black or brown, and *pheomelanin*, which is reddish-yellow. Mixtures of these pigments give different hair colours. Removal of the natural colour, or *bleaching*, is a chemical reaction which changes the pigments to colourless compounds inside the hair shaft. This process takes place by the addition of oxygen to the pigment and the chemical reaction is therefore called *oxidation*.

Black and brown pigments are more easily oxidised than red and yellow pigments, so that the oxidation takes place in three stages:
1. Oxidation of black and brown pigments leaving red and yellow.
2. Oxidation of red pigment leaving yellow.
3. Oxidation of yellow pigment.

The oxygen required for bleaching is usually obtained from the decomposition of hydrogen peroxide, ammonium hydroxide being added as a catalyst to speed the release of oxygen. A *catalyst* is a substance which speeds up a reaction but remains unchanged itself at the end of the reaction. Hydrogen peroxide, because it supplies oxygen for the reaction, is known as an *oxidising agent*.

Hydrogen peroxide ⟶ oxygen + water

Newly formed oxygen or *nascent* (new-born) *oxygen* is a powerful bleaching agent unlike ordinary atmospheric oxygen. The oxidation process of bleaching is represented by the following equation:

Melanin   +   nascent oxygen⟶oxy-melanin
(coloured)   (from hydrogen   (colourless)
                            peroxide)

Experiment 13.1   The preparation of oxygen from hydrogen peroxide. Using the apparatus shown in Fig. 13.1, allow hydrogen peroxide to drop gradually on to the manganese dioxide in the flask. Collect the gas given off in a gas jar, but discard the first jarful as this will contain air. The gas will re-light a glowing splint, and this shows it to be oxygen. Manganese dioxide, a black powder, acts as a catalyst.

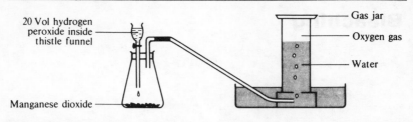

20 Vol hydrogen peroxide inside thistle funnel

Gas jar

Oxygen gas

Water

Manganese dioxide

Fig. 13.1 The preparation of oxygen

Oxides

Hydrogen peroxide is one of a series of compounds called *oxides*. An oxide is formed by the combination of any single element with oxygen.

Element + oxygen ⟶ an oxide

Many oxides (though not hydrogen peroxide) are formed by burning elements in oxygen.

Acidic oxides are formed if non-metal elements such as carbon or sulphur are burned in oxygen. These oxides produce acids when they dissolve in water.

Example:
Carbon + oxygen → carbon dioxide
Carbon dioxide + water → carbonic acid
Acidic oxide + water → an acid

Basic oxides are formed when metal elements such as sodium and calcium are burned in oxygen. If they dissolve in water an alkali (a hydroxide) is produced.

Example:
sodium + oxygen → sodium oxide
Sodium oxide + water → sodium hydroxide
Basic oxide + water → an alkali

Neutral oxides such as water are neither basic nor acidic. If hydrogen is burned in oxygen, water is produced. Each molecule of water contains two atoms of hydrogen and one atom of oxygen, and is represented by the chemical formula H_2O.

Peroxides such as hydrogen peroxide and magnesium peroxide will give off oxygen on heating, and contain a greater proportion of oxygen than other oxides. Each molecule of hydrogen peroxide contains two atoms of hydrogen combined with two atoms of oxygen, and is represented by the formula H_2O_2.

Experiment 13.2   Preparation and classification of oxides.
Using the apparatus for Experiment 13.1, collect several jars of oxygen, and using deflagrating spoons burn a different element in each jar. Add

a little water to dissolve the oxide formed and test the solution with litmus paper. Suitable elements and typical results are shown in Table 13.1. The experiment shows that the oxides formed from non-metal elements produce acid solutions, and the oxides from metal elements produce alkaline solutions.

Table 13.1 Formation of oxides.

Element	Type	Oxide formed	Effect on litmus of a solution of the oxide
Sodium	Metal	Sodium oxide	Turns blue (alkaline)
Magnesium	Metal	Magnesium oxide	Turns blue (alkaline)
Carbon	Non-metal	Carbon dioxide	Turns red (acid)
Phosphorus	Non-metal	Phosphorus oxide	Turns red (acid)
Sulphur	Non-metal	Sulphur dioxide	Turns red (acid)

The properties of hydrogen peroxide

1. Hydrogen peroxide is a colourless liquid.
2. For salon use, hydrogen peroxide is available in various 'volume strengths' from 10 volume to 100 volume. *The volume strength* is the number of parts of free oxygen obtainable from one part of the hydrogen peroxide.

   Thus: 1 part of 20 volume hydrogen peroxide gives 20 parts of free oxygen; or 1 ml of 20 volume hydrogen peroxide gives 20 ml of free oxygen, or 1 ml of 100 volume hydrogen peroxide gives 100 ml of free oxygen.

The strength of hydrogen peroxide may also be expressed as the percentage of pure hydrogen peroxide in the solution. *The percentage strength* is the number of grams of hydrogen peroxide in a hundred grams of solution. Thus a 30 per cent solution contains 30 g of hydrogen peroxide, and therefore 70 g of water in 100 g of solution. As 1 ml of 30 per cent solution of hydrogen peroxide gives 100 ml of free oxygen, a 30 per cent solution is equivalent to a 100 volume strength solution. The percentage strength corresponding to other volume strengths are calculated by proportion.

100 volume strength	=	30% solution
10 volume strength	=	3% solution
20 volume strength	=	6% solution
30 volume strength	=	9% solution
40 volume strength	=	12% solution
60 volume strength	=	18% solution

The volume strength is measured by a special type of hydrometer (see page 187) called a *peroxometer* (see Fig. 13.2). This is floated in hydrogen peroxide and the volume strength is read directly on the scale at surface level.

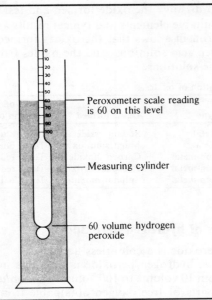

Peroxometer scale reading is 60 on this level

Measuring cylinder

60 volume hydrogen peroxide

Fig. 13.2 Use of a peroxometer

Experiment 13.3   To find the volume strength of hydrogen peroxide. An approximate value of the volume strength may be obtained by direct measurement, using the apparatus shown in Fig. 13.3. Fill the burette with 20 volume hydrogen peroxide and allow 1 ml of it to drop gradually on to the manganese dioxide in the flask. Measure the number of millilitres of oxygen produced, by collecting the oxygen in a measuring cylinder inverted over water and noting the reading of the water surface in the cylinder.

1 ml of 20 volume hydrogen peroxide should give 20 ml of oxygen. Repeat the experiment using 40 volume hydrogen peroxide.

1 ml of 40 volume hydrogen peroxide should give 40 ml of oxygen.

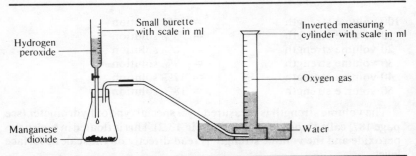

Small burette with scale in ml

Hydrogen peroxide

Inverted measuring cylinder with scale in ml

Oxygen gas

Manganese dioxide

Water

Fig. 13.3 To determine the volume strength of hydrogen peroxide

3. Hydrogen peroxide is an *oxidising agent* as it gives oxygen to other substances during chemical reactions. Concentrated hydrogen peroxide may break the polypeptide chains in hair keratin by oxidation so causing breakage of the hair shaft. It also causes skin burns. Forty volume hydrogen peroxide is the strongest solution which can be applied to hair without damage.

   In hairdressing, hydrogen peroxide is used as follows:
   (a) as an oxidising bleach (20–30 volume for normal bleaching and 40 volume for bleached tips);
   (b) for the oxidation of permanent dyes (10–30 volume);
   (c) as an oxidising agent in perming (20 volume).

4. Hydrogen peroxide is easily decomposed into water and oxygen by the following:
   (a) alkalis such as ammonium hydroxide;   (b) heat from the sun or radiators;   (c) sunlight;   (d) dust;   (e) copper, lead or iron compounds;   (f) organic substances such as blood.

5. Acids tend to prevent the decomposition of hydrogen peroxide and are often used as *stabilisers* added during manufacture to prevent loss of oxygen during storage. Small quantities of salicylic acid or phosphoric acid are used for this purpose.

The storage of hydrogen peroxide

Since hydrogen peroxide is easily decomposed, it should be protected from substances and conditions which lead to its decomposition:

1. It should be stored in a cool dark place, preferably in a dark bottle though this is not essential if the peroxide is stabilised.
2. The stopper should be replaced immediately after use and kept tightly in place, to prevent the entry of dust.
3. Storage bottles should be smooth on the inside, as any projection forms a point at which decomposition begins.
4. As with other chemicals, hydrogen peroxide once poured out should not be returned to the bottle.
5. Hydrogen peroxide, though not itself flammable, assists fire by giving off oxygen when heated. Consequently it should not be stored near flammable liquids such as alcohol or lacquer sprays.
6. It should be stored in relatively small quantities to prevent deterioration during its shelf life. The more concentrated the hydrogen peroxide, the more liable is it to lose its strength.

The dilution of hydrogen peroxide

If the correct volume strength of hydrogen peroxide is not available it is sometimes necessary to dilute a stock solution of a higher strength to obtain the required lower strength solution. Since tap water may be slightly alkaline and would therefore decompose the hydrogen peroxide, dilution should be carried out when necessary by using de-ionised water. The quantity of water to be added for the dilution may be calculated as shown in the following examples.

1. To obtain 30 volume hydrogen peroxide from 60 volume:
   30 volume hydrogen peroxide is $^{30}/_{60}$ or $^1/_2$ as strong as 60 volume. Therefore $^1/_2$ the diluted solution must be 60 volume hydrogen peroxide and the remainder ($^1/_2$) is water.
   Or the solution contains equal quantities of 60 volume hydrogen peroxide and water.

2. To obtain 20 volume hydrogen peroxide from 60 volume:
   20 volume hydrogen peroxide is $^{20}/_{60}$ or $^1/_3$ as strong as 60 volume. Therefore $^1/_3$ of the diluted solution must be 60 volume hydrogen peroxide and the remainder ($^2/_3$) is water.
   Or the solution contains 1 part of hydrogen peroxide to 2 parts of water.

3. To obtain 30 volume hydrogen peroxide from 40 volume:
   30 volume hydrogen peroxide is $^{30}/_{40}$ or $^3/_4$ as strong as 40 volume. Therefore $^3/_4$ of the diluted solution must be 40 volume hydrogen peroxide and the remainder ($^1/_4$) is water.
   Or the solution contains 3 parts of 40 volume hydrogen peroxide to 1 part of water.

Other dilutions are listed in Table 13.2

Table 13.2   Dilution of hydrogen peroxide by volume strength

Stock solution	Required solution	Fraction of stock hydrogen peroxide required	Therefore fraction of water	Proportion hydrogen : water peroxide
100 vol	To 60 vol	$^{60}/_{100} = ^3/_5$	$^2/_5$	3 : 2
100 vol	To 40 vol	$^{40}/_{100} = ^2/_5$	$^3/_5$	2 : 3
100 vol	To 30 vol	$^{30}/_{100} = ^3/_{10}$	$^7/_{10}$	3 : 7
100 vol	To 20 vol	$^{20}/_{100} = ^2/_{10} = ^1/_5$	$^4/_5$	1 : 4
60 vol	To 40 vol	$^{40}/_{60} = ^2/_3$	$^1/_3$	2 : 1
40 vol	To 30 vol	$^{30}/_{40} = ^3/_4$	$^1/_4$	3 : 1
40 vol	To 20 vol	$^{20}/_{40} = ^1/_2$	$^1/_2$	1 : 1
30 vol	To 20 vol	$^{20}/_{30} = ^2/_3$	$^1/_3$	2 : 1

Dilutions involving percentage strengths instead of volume strengths are calculated in the same way (see Table 13.3).

Table 13.3   Dilution of hydrogen peroxide by percentage strength

Stock solution (%)	Required solution (%)	Fraction of stock hydrogen peroxide required	Therefore fraction of water	Proportion hydrogen : water peroxide
30	6	$^6/_{30} = ^1/_5$	$^4/_5$	1 : 4
18	6	$^6/_{18} = ^1/_3$	$^2/_3$	1 : 2
12	3	$^3/_{12} = ^1/_4$	$^3/_4$	1 : 3
30	12	$^{12}/_{30} = ^2/_5$	$^3/_5$	2 : 3

The use of ammonium hydroxide in bleaching

Ammonium hydroxide is an alkali formed when ammonia gas dissolves in water. By itself it has no bleaching power. When added to hydrogen peroxide used for bleaching, ammonium hydroxide has the following functions:

(a) to neutralise the acid stabiliser in the hydrogen peroxide;
(b) to open the cuticle scales to allow easy penetration of the bleach into the hair shaft;
(c) to act as a wetting agent;
(d) to act as a catalyst to speed the release of oxygen from the hydrogen peroxide.

The strongest ammonium hydroxide solution obtainable contains 35 per cent of ammonia gas dissolved in water, and readily gives off choking fumes of ammonia gas, so that it must be used with care. It should be stored in a cool place to prevent decomposition and loss of ammonia. This strong solution is often referred to as '0·880 ammonia', the figure 0·880 being the *relative density* (specific gravity) of the solution.

The relative density of a substance is the number of times the substance is as heavy as an equal volume of water.

$$\text{Relative density} = \frac{\text{the mass of a substance}}{\text{the mass of an equal volume of water}}$$

Ammonium hydroxide with a relative density of 0·880 weighs 0·880 times as much as an equal volume of water.

The relative density of a liquid is measured by means of a *hydrometer* (see Fig. 13.4), which is floated in the liquid, and the relative density is

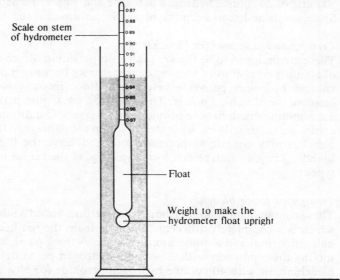

Scale on stem of hydrometer

0·87
0·88
0·89
0·90
0·91
0·92
0·93
0·94
0·95
0·96
0·97

Float

Weight to make the hydrometer float upright

Fig. 13.4 Measuring the relative density of a liquid

read directly at surface level on the scale of the stem of the instrument. A hydrometer always displaces the same weight of liquid. If the relative density of the liquid is small, a greater volume will be displaced, so the hydrometer will sink low in the liquid. Similarly the hydrometer will float high to displace a small volume of a dense liquid.

The relative density of water is 1 and if 0·880 ammonium hydroxide loses its strength, its relative density will increase to approach that of water. A hydrometer with a scale graduated between 0·880 and 1 can thus be used to measure the strength of ammonium hydroxide solution.

The composition of bleaches

Bleaching preparations contain two parts which are mixed immediately before use.
1. **An oxidising agent**, usually hydrogen peroxide or magnesium peroxide, to provide nascent oxygen for bleaching.
2. **An alkaline substance**, usually ammonium hydroxide solution or solid ammonium carbonate, to release the oxygen from hydrogen peroxide by acting as a catalyst. The alkali gives a pH of 8–9.5 and causes the hair to swell.

Types of bleach

Simple liquid bleach
This is used as a brightening shampoo to revive blonde hair which has darkened with age or to give highlights to light brown hair. It contains 50 parts of 20 volume hydrogen peroxide and 1 part of 0·880 ammonia. Shampoo is added to keep the bleach in position on the hair.

Cream, emulsion and oil bleaches
These are designed to be thicker than a simple liquid bleach and consist of alkaline emulsions of various consistencies. They are mixed with 20 volume hydrogen peroxide before use. Boosters may be added to increase the bleaching power. These contain potassium persulphate or ammonium persulphate to provide extra oxygen. Conditioners such as cetrimide are usually incorporated to lessen the damage to the hair. Oil bleaches may contain sulphonated oils and leave the hair a golden blonde. They do not bleach as completely as the cream or emulsion types.

Powder or paste bleaches
These contain magnesium carbonate (sometimes called white henna but which is a completely different substance from the red henna used in hair colouring) and ammonium carbonate. A thick paste is formed by mixing these powders with 20 volume hydrogen peroxide for general bleaching, or with 40 volume hydrogen peroxide for bleached streaks

and tips. This type of bleach is the most powerful used in hairdressing, and may leave the hair rough and porous.

Gel bleaches
Many modern bleaches are of this type. The gelling agent acts as a thickener of the bleach. Lauryl diethanolamide is often used and gels on addition of hydrogen peroxide. If boosters are added, carbopol may be used as the gelling agent.

To increase the speed of bleaching

Damage to the hair during bleaching is decreased if contact time with the bleach is reduced, so heat is applied to speed the chemical reaction. The heat may be moist heat applied by use of a steamer or dry heat by use of infra-red lamps.

The *steamer* consists basically of an electric kettle with a hood to direct steam slowly over the client's head (see Fig. 13.5). De-ionised water should be used in the steamer to prevent loss of efficiency, by the accumulation of salts produced as 'scale' from temporary hard water or left in the steamer after the evaporation of permanently hard water.

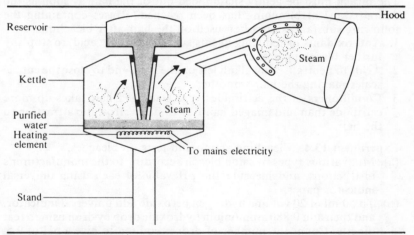

Fig. 13.5 A steamer

Infra-red heat is applied by use of *an accelerator* containing about 100 small 5 watt lamps, which are arranged in banks with separate control switches. The machine has a three-heat switch to control the intensity of radiation, and a time switch. Other models contain only ten to twelve lamps of higher wattage. Infra-red lamps of 275 watts are also mounted in groups of three or five on a stand, each lamp being attached to a flexible metal arm so that the lamps can be positioned as required. In contrast to the moist heat of the steamer, infra-red lamps give a dry heat which tends to dry out the bleach and terminate the bleaching process if not carefully controlled.

Cause of damage to the hair during bleaching

Breakage of the hair during bleaching may be caused by:
1. Overbleaching, either by use of too strong hydrogen peroxide or too long processing time. The breakage occurs due to splitting of the polypeptide chains of amino acids by oxidation.
2. The use of bleaches with too high pH values. Strong alkalis soften and finally destroy hair. The pH value should be less than 9·5.
3. The overlapping of previously bleached portions of the hair when bleaching a regrowth.

   Damage to the cuticle may also result from over bleaching. The hair may be left spongy and porous with a tendency to retain moisture on subsequent washing and become difficult to dry out. The cuticle may be left roughened or in some cases the cuticle scales may actually be destroyed.

Treatment when bleaching is completed

The bleach must be gently shampooed out of the hair as soon as the desired stage of bleaching has been reached. Rinses containing the following substances are often used on the hair after bleaching:
1. **Anti-oxidants** or reducing agents such as ascorbic acid, to stop any further bleaching action.
2. **Acids** to neutralise any alkali left on the hair, and to close the cuticle scales making the hair smoother.
3. **Conditioners** of the cetrimide type. Damaged hair takes up more cetrimide than undamaged hair due to its electrostatic attraction to the hair.

Experiment 13.4   Bleaching action and tests on bleaches.
(a) Mix various types of salon bleach according to the manufacturer's instructions, and measure the pH value of each using universal indicator paper.
(b) To 50 ml of 20 volume hydrogen peroxide add universal indicator, and then add 0·880 ammonium hydroxide drop by drop using a teat pipette. Count the number of drops required to give a pH of 9·5, and compare this amount with the amount used in a simple liquid bleach.
(c) Obtain a sample of dark hair (8–10 cm in length), and prepare four small bundles. Place each bundle in a separate test tube and add the following:
   To test tube (1) 21 ml of purified water (control).
                 (2) 20 ml purified water and 1 ml 0·88 ammonia.
                 (3) 20 ml 20 volume of hydrogen peroxide and 1 ml of purified water.
                 (4) 20 ml of 20 volume hydrogen peroxide and 1 ml of 0·88 ammonia.

Leave the samples in a water bath at 37°C for about half an hour and note the tube in which bleaching takes place. Deduce which substances cause bleaching.

(d) Compare the bleaching powers of different strengths of hydrogen peroxide as follows:

Prepare four bundles of dark brown hair (8–10 cm in length) and place them in separate test tubes. Add a different strength of hydrogen peroxide (20, 30, 40 and 60 volume) to each sample, along with a few drops of 0·880 ammonia. Leave the tubes in a water bath at 37°C for half an hour to allow bleaching to take place. Compare the amount of bleaching in each case. Repeat using different shades of hair in 20 volume hydrogen peroxide.

(e) Over-bleach a sample of hair by applying a strong paste bleach and keeping it at 37°C for 30 minutes. Wash the sample and note the texture by touch and by examination through a microscope. Compare the sample with the original hair.

Questions

1. Explain what is meant by:
   (a) an acid;   (b) an alkali.
   Describe the effect of acids on:
   (a) hair;   (b) hydrogen peroxide.
   Describe the effect of alkalis on:
   (a) hair;   (b) hydrogen peroxide.
2. A supply of 40 volume hydrogen peroxide and some de-ionised water are available.
   Explain how you would obtain the following:
   (a) 20 ml of 30 volume hydrogen peroxide;
   (b) 30 ml of 20 volume hydrogen peroxide;
   (c) 40 ml of 10 volume hydrogen peroxide.
3. What precautions should be taken to avoid damage to hair during bleaching?
4. Explain the meaning of:
   (a) nascent oxygen;   (b) a wetting agent;   (c) an emulsion;
   (d) an oxide.
   Give examples in each case.
5. Explain fully why:
   (a) hydrogen peroxide should not be used in a metal dish;
   (b) forty volume peroxide may be used for bleached tips but not on a full head;
   (c) hydrogen peroxide should not be poured out into a dish until required:
   (d) any unused hydrogen peroxide should not be poured back into the storage bottle.

Chapter 14

Hair colouring

The colouring of hair is achieved by the application of a pigment or a mixture of pigments, in the form of a dye. Unless some bleaching is taking place at the same time, colouring involves the addition of the dye to the natural pigment of the hair. Thus the natural colour must always be taken into consideration before dyeing. The pigment in hair, whether natural or applied, produces colour by absorbing certain wavelengths or colours of light, and allowing others to be reflected to our eyes. A pigment thus *subtracts* colours from the white daylight or artificial light falling on it. The light which is reflected gives the colour we see, and the pigment is named by that reflected colour. Thus if red light is reflected we say that the pigment is red. When pigments are mixed, each pigment subtracts its own band of colour from the white light leaving fewer colours to be reflected. If all the colours are absorbed by an object it appears black, as no light is reflected. The mixing of pigments therefore tends towards the production of black. Both the application of dyes to hair and the manufacture of dyes themselves involve the mixing of pigments.

Mixing pigments

In practice, pigments rarely reflect one single spectrum colour, but reflect varying amounts of a band of adjacent spectrum colours. The order of colours in the spectrum is red, orange, yellow, green, blue and violet. Thus a yellow pigment normally reflects orange and green in addition to yellow, whilst a blue pigment also reflects a little green and violet (see Fig. 14.1). If yellow and blue pigments are mixed, the only colour reflected by both is green, since the mixture strongly absorbs the other spectrum colours (see Fig. 14.2).

Adding red pigments to the mixture of yellow and blue will result in the absorption of the green (see Fig. 14.3). No colour will therefore be reflected, and so the mixture produces black. This is only true if the pigments in the mixture are present in the correct proportion. Different proportions of the three pigments may produce brown or grey. Manufacturers obtain many shades of brown in semi-permanent and temporary dyes by mixing red, blue and yellow pigments in different proportions.

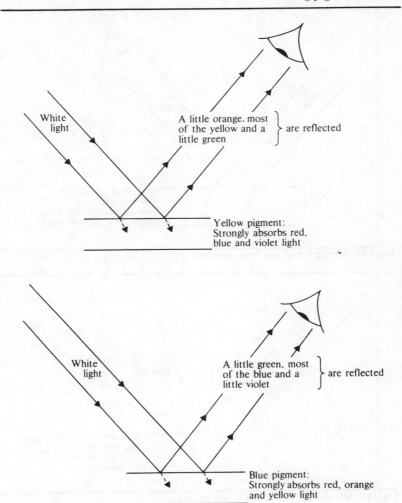

Fig. 14.1 Reflection of light by pigments

Adding colour to the hair may result in the development of *unwanted colours*, particularly if the hair is blonde and contains yellow pigment; or if the hair is grey and contains a mixture of coloured and white hairs. Consider the effect of adding auburn (red) dye to various types of hair. Added to brown hair, the dye would produce an acceptable red-brown; but added to blonde (yellow) it would result in orange (yellow + red = orange). Similarly, added to grey hair (a mixture of light brown and white) the brown would become red-brown (acceptable) but white would become red (unacceptable).

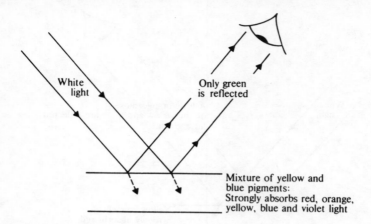

Fig. 14.2 Mixing yellow and blue pigments

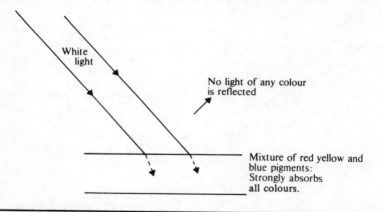

Fig. 14.3 Mixing red, yellow and blue pigments

Adding a blue rinse or an ash colour which may contain blue pigment to blonde (yellow) hair may give rise to an unwanted green cast (blue + yellow = green). The unwanted colour may be corrected by the addition of a small quantity of a suitable pigment which will absorb the offending colour. Thus a little red pigment will absorb green, or a green dye (some ash shades contain green pigment) will absorb red.

A colour triangle of the spectrum colours is shown in Fig. 14.4, and is useful as an aid to colour correction. The offending colour may be corrected by addition of the colour opposite to it in the colour triangle.

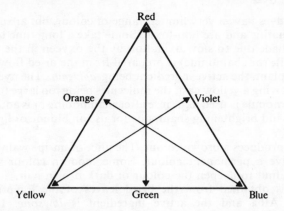

Fig. 14.4 The colour triangle

The qualities of a good dye

A good dye should
1. Not damage the hair or cause irritation of the skin.
2. Not be toxic.
3. Be quick in action.
4. Be easy to apply.
5. Give a natural looking colour.
6. Not fade with time or by the action of sunlight.
7. Be unaffected by later processing such as bleaching or perming.

No hair colouring agents possess all these qualities but modern permanent dyes give a most reliable colour, though they tend to cause dermatitis and some are suspected of causing cancer. Natural vegetable dyes are safest but have many other disadvantages.

Types of dye

Hair dyes are classified into the following groups:
1. Natural vegetable dyes which include henna, walnut and camomile.
2. Metallic dyes such as sulphide dyes.
3. Synthetic dyes which are subdivided into:
   (a) oxidation or para dyes which only reach their final colour by oxidation inside the hair shaft;
   (b) direct dyes which are applied in their final form and include:
       (i) semi-permanent dyes or nitro dyes;
       (ii) temporary dyes such as azo dyes.

Vegetable dyes

Vegetable dyes have a very limited range of colour, but are unlikely to cause dermatitis and are non-toxic. Some take a long time to develop the final shade due to slow oxidation by the oxygen in the air.

Camomile (or chamomile) is prepared from the dried flowers of the camomile plant, the active ingredient being *apigenin*. The dye coats the hair shaft giving a yellow cast, the molecules being too large to enter the cortex. Camomile is used as a rinse after shampooing or is added to hair lightening and brightening shampoos for use on blonde or light brown hair.

Walnut produces a brown colour. The juice of unripe walnut shells is used to give a permanent colour. Some modern colour shampoos contain walnut to deepen the colour of dark brown hair.

Henna is obtained from the dried leaves of the Egyptian privet Lawsonia Alba and the active ingredient is *lawsone*. It gives a permanent colour by penetrating the hair shaft to produce red shades, which may be emphasised by the addition of acetic acid or made slightly browner by the addition of borax (alkaline). The dye is progressive as it is oxidised slowly by the oxygen in the air, and takes about two days to reach its final shade. If the leaves are collected before fully mature the product is known as *Green Henna*, and this gives a more delicate shade of red than normal henna. Indigo, from the plant of that name, used to be mixed with henna to produce *Persian Henna* or *Henna Reng*, which dyed hair a magnificent blue-black colour. Modern colour shampoos may contain henna to give auburn highlights to brown and chestnut hair. It is also used as a dye on black hair and gives an attractive red cast, particularly in bright sunlight.

Metallic dyes

Inorganic salts are used in *'hair colour restorers'*. Lead salts or silver salts applied to the hair gradually darken by the action of hydrogen sulphide in the air, and so 'restore' hair colour. The effect may be increased by the addition of sodium thiosulphate to the salts.

In *two-application dyes*, or 'sulphide dyes', the hair is first treated with sodium sulphide solution and then with the solution of a metallic salt such as lead acetate, silver nitrate or copper sulphate. Double decomposition takes place and a metal sulphide is deposited both in the cortex and on the surface of the hair.

For example:

sodium sulphide + copper sulphate → sodium sulphate + copper sulphide
(black)

Metallic dyes have many disadvantages.
1. Some, such as lead and copper salts, are poisonous.
2. They give a dull appearance to the hair.
3. Strong sodium sulphide is a depilatory (hair remover).

4. It is difficult to perm hair which has previously been treated with metallic dyes, since the chemicals used in perming may react with the dye. Copper and iron salts may act as catalysts, causing the vigorous decomposition of hydrogen peroxide (used in 'neutraliser' during perming) with resulting hair breakage.

Experiment 14.1   The preparation of sulphide dyes.
Prepare the following solutions:
0·5 g of sodium sulphide in 100 ml of water;
2 g of silver nitrate in 100 ml of water;
2 g of lead acetate in 100 ml of water;
1 g of copper sulphate in 100 ml of water.

Immerse three wefts of blonde or bleached hair in sodium sulphide solution and then immediately transfer one weft to each of the other solutions. Note the colour produced. Shampoo and then dry the hair to test the permanence of the dye.

Experiment 14.2   The effect of sodium sulphide on hair.
Leave a weft of hair immersed in sodium sulphide solution for a short time. Notice softening and disintegration of the hair.

Experiment 14.3   To test hair for metallic salts before perming.
If it is suspected that hair has been treated with a metallic 'hair colour restorer', cut a strand from the hair and immerse it in 20 volume hydrogen peroxide. Bubbles of oxygen will appear and heat will be produced if metallic hair dyes have been used.

Compound henna consists of a mixture of henna and silver, copper or lead salts. A typical formula is:

Henna	72 g
pyrogallic acid	12 g
copper sulphate	8 g
burnt sienna	8 g

The ingredients are mixed to a paste with water at about 70°C before use. The presence of metallic dyes make these preparations poisonous, and it is also difficult to perm the hair afterwards.

Synthetic organic dyes

These form the most modern and widely used group of dyes. They are based on coal tar products such as aniline and consist of oxidation dyes and direct dyes.

1. Oxidation dyes
The earliest oxidation dyes were para-phenylenediamine (diamino-benzene) which produced a black compound on oxidation, and para-toluenediamine (diamino-toluene) which produced a brown compound.

The series of dyes thus became known as para dyes. A large number of other chemicals have now been added to the series to give a wider range of colours. These include:

para-aminophenol (reddish brown)
meta-dihydroxybenzene (grey)
meta-phenylenediamine (brown)

Mixtures of these dyes are prepared as thick liquids or creams designed to be mixed with 20-volume hydrogen peroxide immediately before use. The following substances are added to the mixture of dyes during manufacture.

(a) ammonium hydroxide (producing a pH of about 9) to raise the cuticle scales and allow easy penetration of the dye molecules, and to catalyse the decomposition of the hydrogen peroxide, so releasing oxygen;

(b) sodium sulphite (a reducing agent) to prevent premature oxidation of the dye;

(c) conditioners such as lanolin and cetyl alcohol;

(d) foaming agents such as triethanolamine soaps, to facilitate rinsing off the excess dye.

The final colour of the dye is only reached by oxidation, which takes place inside the hair shaft. The small colourless dye molecules enter the cortex along with hydrogen peroxide. On oxidation, large coloured molecules are formed which become trapped in the hair shaft as they are too large to wash out (see Fig. 14.5). The dye thus produces a permanent colour, but the periodic dyeing of the new-growth of hair is essential if the colour is to be maintained.

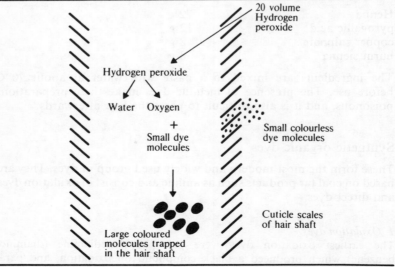

Fig. 14.5 Permanent colour

| small colourless dye molecules | + | oxygen from hydrogen peroxide | → | large coloured molecules which become trapped in the cortex |

The oxidation reaction is slow and may take 10 to 30 minutes to complete, but the dye should not be mixed with hydrogen peroxide until required for use, as any large molecules formed would not then be able to enter the hair shaft. On the hair, oxidation may be speeded by heat from a steamer, an accelerator or infra-red heater.

Replacing 20 volume hydrogen peroxide by the 30 volume strength enables bleaching and dyeing to take place at the same time, and the hair may be dyed lighter than the natural shade.

A rinse containing antioxidants (reducing agents) and acid is beneficial after the excess colour has been rinsed off, to stop the action of the hydrogen peroxide, to neutralise any alkaline substance left on the hair and to close the cuticle scales. Ascorbic acid, which is both a reducing agent and an acid, is often used for this purpose.

Advantages.   Para-dyes are easy to use, and have a good range of natural looking colours. Under normal conditions little or no fading takes place, and there is no difficulty if the hair is permed later, though perms may result in a slight loss of colour.

Disadvantages.   A serious disadvantage of para-dyes is the danger of *dye dermatitis*. A small proportion of people are allergic to the dye. By law, all dyes containing para-phenylenediamine or para-toluenediamine must be labelled to state the percentage content. In some countries use of these substances is restricted.

The mildest symptoms of dye dermatitis are a slight itching and redness of the skin round the hair line. More severe symptoms may include the swelling of the whole face, the developments of papules and general prostration. A client who has been using the dye over a long period may suddenly develop a sensitivity to the dye, so it is essential to give a skin test before each application. The usual test is the *Sabouraud – Rousseau test* (also called a predisposition or hyper-sensitivity test) which is carried out as follows:

Using surgical spirit clean a small area of skin (the size of a 5p coin) either behind the ear close to the hair line or on the inside of the elbow. Mix a little of the required dye with 20 volume hydrogen peroxide and apply a drop to the cleaned area. Allow the dye to dry, and then cover it with a protective layer of collodion. Leave for 24 hours. If any irritation or redness occurs, however slight, the dye should not be applied to the hair. The area may be treated with calamine lotion to relieve the irritation.

Precautions during use.
(a) Always give a skin test 24 hours before applying the dye;
(b) Hairdressers should always wear protective gloves when using para-dyes, not only to prevent staining the hands but also to avoid dermatitis;

(c) The dye should never be applied to eyelashes and eyebrows;
(d) The dye should never be allowed to enter a cut.

Removal of unwanted dye.   If, due to a mistake, it is necessary to remove oxidation dyes from the hair, reducing agents such as sodium formaldehyde sulphoxylate or a 5 per cent solution of sodium bisulphite may be used.

Experiment 14.4   To compare the colour on various shades of hair produced by use of an oxidation dye.
Using small quantities of salon dyes mixed with 20 volume hydrogen peroxide, treat bundles of differently coloured hair about 10 cm in length (use of dark brown, light brown, blonde and grey hair) with the same colour of dye. Place the dyed strands on a watch glass over a water bath at 40°C for 30 minutes. Always wear rubber gloves and use a brush for application. Wash the strands and note the variation in colour. Repeat, using different dyes.

2. Direct dyes
Direct dyes are already coloured in their final form when applied to the hair and do not require oxidation. They include semi-permanent dyes which last through six to eight shampoos, and temporary dyes which are washed out at the first shampoo.
Semi-permanent colours. Semi-permanent colours often consist of nitro-dyes such as nitro-phenylenediamine (nitro-diamino-benzene) which gives red and yellow colours, and anthraquinones which give blue colours. Various mixtures of these three colours will produce a wide range of different shades.

   The molecules are small enough to enter the hair shaft, where they partly combine with the hydrogen bonds in keratin. Each time the hair is washed, water replaces some of the dye molecules in the bonds and the dye gradually washes out.

   The dye mixture is made alkaline (pH 8 to 9) to aid penetration into the cortex, and quaternary ammonium compounds are added to give an even distribution of colour.

   Semi-permanent dyes may be removed by the use of spirit soap (four parts of soft soap dissolved in one part of industrial methylated spirit).

   Some so called semi-permanent dyes or quasi-permanent dyes are mixtures of semi-permanent and oxidation dyes, and require the addition of hydrogen peroxide. These dyes should be regarded as permanent dyes and the same precautions taken as for oxidation dyes. Since the semi-permanent part of the dye washes out there is a gradual loss of colour, but the loss is not complete due to the presence of oxidation dyes, so there is a problem of regrowth.

Temporary colours.   Temporary dyes have molecules which are too large to enter the cortex, so they merely coat the hair shaft. There are various forms of temporary dye but all wash out at the first shampoo.

(i)   **Colour rinses** are used after shampooing and are allowed to dry on the hair. They are intended to cover grey, bleached or white hair. They may contain basic dyes such as methylene blue and methyl violet, which cling to the acid groups in the hair. More often however, they are formulated with such acid dyes (azo dyes) as para-hydroxyazo benzene (yellow) and phenylazonaphthol (red). Organic acids such as citric acid or tartaric acid are added to make the dye cling to the hair shaft.

(ii) **Coloured setting lotions** contain acid dyes added to a plastic film former, which is dissolved in alcohol and water. A coloured plastic film is left on the hair shaft after drying (see Chapter 11 on 'Setting the hair').

(iii) **Coloured lacquers** also contain azo dyes together with plastic resin dissolved in alcohol. The lacquer is sprayed on to the hair after dressing out. Finely powdered aluminium may be added to some lacquers to give a silver lustre.

(iv) **Colour shampoos** may contain synthetic azo dyes added to the detergent along with organic acids such as citric acid or lactic acid to give a pH value of about 5. The shampoos do not produce a marked change in hair colour but brighten faded hair and add highlights.

Experiment 14.5   To separate the colours in commercial plastic setting lotions by chromatography.
Make up a solvent containing:

butanol	100 ml
0·880 ammonia	1 ml
water	44 ml
ethanol	20 ml

Place 50 ml of this solvent in a Shandon chromatography tank. Drop a spot of each of six different colours of setting lotions on a chromatography paper (25 cm by 25 cm) about 2 cm from the bottom of the paper as shown in Fig. 14.6. Clip the sides of the paper together to form a cylinder, and stand the paper in the solvent inside the tank, ensuring that the spots of dye are above the level of the solvent. The solvent travels up the paper by capillary rise, separating the colours in the setting lotions due to differences in their solubility. The most soluble of the mixture of dyes will travel highest up the paper. If a Shandon tank is not available, strips of chromatography paper may be suspended from a cork in a measuring cylinder or boiling tube. When separation has taken place, allow the paper to dry in a fume cupboard. Note the colours produced from each dye. Brown dyes will be found to consist of various proportions of the three pigments red, blue and yellow.

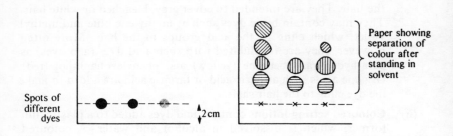

Fig. 14.6 Separation of colours by chromatography

Questions

1. What is meant by oxidation?
   List the hairdressing processes which involve oxidation and explain the reaction in each case.
2. Explain the procedure you would adopt if:
   (a) a client's hair developed an unwanted green cast;
   (b) you suspected that a client requiring a perm had been using a metallic 'hair colour restorer';
   (c) a client's skin became inflamed after a test with para-dye.
3. What are the properties of cetrimide?
   In what hairdressing preparations is cetrimide (or other similar quaternary ammonium compound) used?
4. What is the meaning of:
   (a) non-toxic dyes;   (b) double decomposition;   (c) an allergy;
   (d) capillary rise.
   Give examples in each case.
5. What is meant by permanent, semi-permanent and temporary hair colours?
   Explain how the size of the molecules in each case affects the action of each type of dye.
   How is it possible to remove an unwanted colour?

Chapter 15

Permanent waving

The reasons for natural curliness or straightness of hair are not fully understood, but ıt is thought that it depends on the shape of the follicle. A straight hair is produced from a straight follicle, and a curly hair from a curved follicle (see Fig. 15.1). The theory that straight hairs have a circular cross section and curly hairs an oval cross section has been discounted. The straightness or curliness of hair may be altered by treating the hair chemically to produce permanent changes in keratin structure. In the permanent waving of hair these chemical changes take place during either cold waving or heat waving. The permanent set so produced cannot be removed by water whatever its temperature.

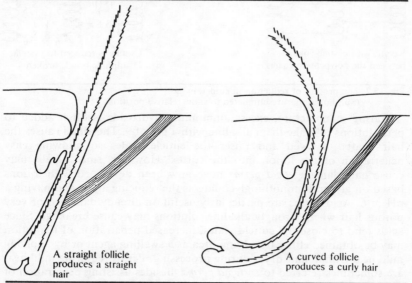

A straight follicle produces a straight hair

A curved follicle produces a curly hair

Fig. 15.1 The effect of follicle shape

Cold permanent waving

During cold waving the hair is wound in sections onto curlers and then undergoes two separate chemical processes.

1.   Chemical reduction

The lotion applied to the hair in the first process of cold waving is a solution containing ammonium thioglycollate (ammonium thiolethanoate) though monoethanolamine thioglycollate or ammonium sulphite may also be used. These substances are salts but are also *reducing agents* capable of breaking the disulphide bonds in the keratin of the cortex of the hair. These bonds form part of the cystine linkages which lie between adjacent polypeptide chains in the keratin molecules, and each disulphide bond joins two sulphur atoms. During perming, hydrogen atoms from the reducing agent break some of the disulphide bonds by attaching themselves to the sulphur atoms. The cystine molecules are thus split and each forms two cysteine molecules (see Fig. 15.2). This type of chemical reaction which involves the addition of hydrogen to a substance is called *reduction*.

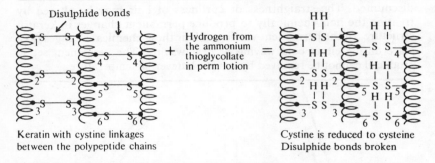

Fig. 15.2 The process of reduction in cold waving
(Sulphur atoms are numbered to show relative positions.)

During manufacture, excess ammonium hydroxide is often added to perm lotions to make them alkaline with a pH of 9. The alkali causes the hair shafts to swell and raises the cuticle scales so allowing easy penetration of the lotion into the cortex. However, since alkalis may cause hair damage, *acid perms* have now been developed with lotions based on glyceryl monothioglycollate as the reducing agent and having a pH of 6. Acid perms are particularly useful on already damaged or very porous hair where strongly alkaline solutions may cause breakage. Since acids tend to close the cuticle scales, increased penetration of the lotion may be obtained either by adding urea as a swelling agent or by applying mild heat from a hair dryer during processing. Perms requiring mild heat are sometimes referred to as *tepid perms*. Besides assisting penetration of the lotion, heat also increases the speed of the chemical reaction so that processing time is reduced. In the case of alkaline lotions, sufficient heat for satisfactory processing is produced if the hair is enclosed in an insulating plastic cap to retain the heat of the scalp.

Whilst keratin is in its reduced state, the hair is fragile and easily broken so must not be subjected to tension. In cold waving the hair must therefore always be wound on to curlers without tension. Breaking the disulphide bonds decreases the number of cross-linkages between the polypeptide chains. This enables the hair to take the physical shape of the curlers by movement of the polypeptide chains in relation to each other (see Fig. 15.3). The firmness of the curl depends on the number of bonds broken and is controlled by the strength of the lotion and the time the lotion is left on the hair. When a satisfactory wave has been produced the lotion must be rinsed from the hair to prevent further reduction from taking place, but the curlers must be left in position until the completion of the oxidation process which follows.

2. Chemical oxidation

The second process of cold waving is carried out to make the newly curled shape permanent, by re-building the disulphide bonds of cystine in a new position on the polypeptide chains. This process is one of *oxidation*, a chemical reaction which involves the addition of oxygen to a substance. (In hairdressing the second process of cold waving is called 'neutralising' but the process involves addition of oxygen and is therefore not chemical neutralisation which is the reaction between an acid and an alkali.) The hair is treated with an *oxidising agent* (called the neutraliser in hairdressing) such as hydrogen peroxide or sodium bromate. Oxygen from the oxidising agent combines with hydrogen in the cysteine molecules to form water. Adjacent sulphur atoms are then able to join together to make new disulphide bonds. Permanent cystine cross linkages are thus formed, so setting the hair in the curled position (see Fig. 15.3). After perming, fewer cross linkages are re-formed than were originally present, therefore perming always involves some weakening of the hair.

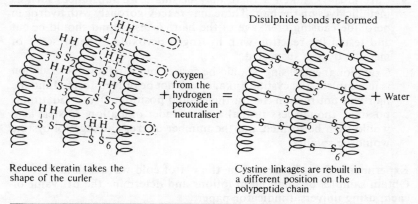

Reduced keratin takes the
shape of the curler

Cystine linkages are rebuilt in
a different position on the
polypeptide chain

Fig. 15.3 The process of oxidation in cold waving
(Sulphur atoms are numbered to show relative positions).

Precautions in cold waving

1. A pre-perm shampoo is necessary to remove sebum from the hair shaft, as this may prevent the penetration of the lotion. A clear

soapless shampoo should be used. Cream shampoos may contain lanolin which would also affect the penetration of the lotion, and soap shampoos may leave a film of lime-soap if the water is hard.

2. The scalp should be inspected for cuts, sores or inflammation and the perm should not be attempted if these are present. Very slight defects may be covered with Vaseline.

3. Perm damage to already porous or over processed hair can be reduced by the use of pre-perm fillers containing protein hydrolysates, which increase bonding in the hair.

4. Perm lotion frequently causes dermatitis. Hairdressers should always wear protective gloves during perming. The lotion should not be allowed to touch the client's skin, and special care should be taken to prevent lotion entering the eyes and ears. Remember that hair, skin and nails are all keratin and if ammonium thioglycollate softens and weakens hair, it will similarly affect the skin and nails.

5. The pH of perm lotion must not be greater than 9·5 or the lotion will damage the hair and may act as a depilatory (a hair remover).

6. The hair should not be pulled or wound too tightly, as perm lotion weakens hair and breakages may occur.

7. Ammonium thioglycollate reacts with iron to form a purple coloured compound. Contact between perm lotion and any iron object should be avoided to prevent discolouration of the hair.

8. The manufacturer's instructions should be carefully read and carried out. In some cases dilution of the lotion is required for bleached and tinted hair, and in other cases several lotions are available, each intended for a different type of hair.

9. Care must be taken if there may be unknown substances such as metallic dyes on the hair. These may react vigorously with hydrogen peroxide causing breakage of the hair. A test strand should be cut and tested for reaction with hydrogen peroxide if the presence of metallic dyes is suspected.

10. Oxidation (neutralising) should be carried out carefully. If oxidation is incomplete, the cystine linkages will not be fully re-formed and the hair will not remain 'set' in the desired position. Over-oxidation is possible, though less probable than under oxidation. Cysteic acid would then be formed and the number of cross linkages of cystine would be smaller.

Experiment 15.1   To determine the pH of cold wave lotions.
Obtain samples of salon perm lotions and determine the pH value of each, using universal indicator paper.

Experiment 15.2   To cold wave a test curl.
(a) Preparation of cold wave lotion by neutralisation of thioglycollic acid by ammonium hydroxide.
Fill a burette with 0·880 ammonium hydroxide which has been diluted with an equal volume of water. Place 20 ml of thioglycollic acid in a conical flask with 20 ml of purified water, and add a few

drops of universal indicator liquid. Gradually add the ammonium hydroxide until the acid is neutralised. The reaction is exothermic (heat is produced). Continue the addition of ammonium hydroxide until the pH is 9. This solution may be used to perm a test curl of cut hair wound on a salon type curler. It must not be used on a client's hair. The test curl should be immersed in the solution for 15 minutes and be kept at about 37°C to represent the warmth of the scalp.

(b) Preparation of neutraliser.

Add 1·5 ml of triethanolamine lauryl sulphate and 5 g of sodium bromate (oxidising agent) to 100 ml of de-ionised water. The triethanolamine lauryl sulphate produces a foam which holds the oxidising mixture on the hair. This solution may be used as a 'neutraliser' for the test curl, after removing it from the perm lotion and rinsing it with cold water. The test curl should be placed in the neutraliser for ten minutes before unwinding, rinsing and drying.

Experiment 15.3   To test the reaction of ammonium thioglycollate on metals.

Dip several small metal objects such as a nail, hair clip, scissors and the metal end of a pin-tail comb into cold wave lotion and rinse them immediately. Note which objects produce a purple compound due to the presence of iron.

Commercial cold wave lotions

Cold wave lotions contain the following ingredients:

1. **A reducing agent** which is usually ammonium thioglycollate, though monoethanolamine thioglycollate may be used. The percentage of reducing agent present determines the use of the lotion. Hair which has had no previous treatment (virgin hair) is difficult to perm and requires a strong lotion containing 10 per cent ammonium thioglycollate. This strength may also be used if a long lasting and tight curl is desired. An 8 per cent solution is suitable for normal hair, and a 5–6 per cent solution for bleached or tinted hair. Glyceryl monothioglycollate is used as the reducing agent in acid perm lotions.
2. **A swelling agent**, usually ammonium hydroxide in alkaline lotions and urea in acid lotions, controls the level of entry of the reducing agent into the cortex.
3. **Conditioners** such as cetrimide, PVP-resins, or protein hydrolysates.
4. **Perfume.** Masking the unpleasant smell of ammonium thioglycollate is difficult as the reducing agent tends to break down the perfume.
5. **Mineral oil and an emulsifying agent** such as cetyl alcohol may be added to form an oil-in-water emulsion which thickens the lotion so that it does not run off the hair.

Commercial neutralisers

The neutraliser may be a cream or a liquid type.

Cream neutralisers consist of an emulsion which is mixed with 20 volume hydrogen peroxide immediately before use.

Liquid types often contain 5 per cent sodium bromate as the oxidising agent and are mixed with 1 per cent soapless detergent solution as a wetting and foaming agent. Citric acid or acetic acid may be added to give a pH of 4. The acid neutralises any alkali left on the hair after perming and closes the cuticle scales, so improving hair condition. Unlike hydrogen peroxide, sodium bromate is effective in acid solution. Sodium bromate reacts explosively with ammonium thioglycollate, therefore neutraliser and perm lotion should never be mixed. Urea may be added to neutraliser as a flame retardant.

Heat permanent waving

Heat perm lotions are solutions of the alkali ammonium hydroxide together with small quantities of a reducing agent such as potassium sulphite or sodium bisulphite which speeds the breakage of the bonds. The lotion is applied to the hair which is then wound fairly tightly on to curlers and heated to about 60°C. The alkali causes bond breaking by hydrolysis and the hair takes the shape of the curler. Hydrolysis means the decomposition of a substance with the addition of the elements of water. As the hair cools, new cross linkages are formed in a different position along the polypeptide chains giving a permanent set. Many of the new bonds are *sulphide bonds* and contain only one sulphur atom. These bonds form part of an amino acid called *lanthionine*. The winding of the curlers may be tighter than in cold waving as the hair is not weakened to the same extent. The re-building of the linkages takes place at the same time as the breakdown process and not as a separate reaction as in cold waving.

The heat may be applied by the following methods:

1. **Electrical heaters** attached to each curl (early method).
2. **Steam processing** (early method).
3. **Hot metal clips** heated by conduction from electric elements on a wire-less or falling-heat machine. A heated clip is placed over each curl, the scalp being insulated by rubber pads to prevent burns.
   In the modern equivalent of this method plastic clips are used and heated in a similar way but to a lower temperature.
4. **Exothermic pads** containing calcium oxide (quicklime). When the pad is wetted, heat is produced by the following reaction:

Calcium oxide + water ⟶ calcium hydroxide + heat
(a basic oxide)   (an alkali)

Since heat is given out, this reaction is said to be exothermic. The water-saturated pads or sachets are clipped one to each curl and left in position until cold. The sachets become hot enough to burn the client's skin so they must not be allowed to touch the scalp. The sachets should not be opened, as chemical burns would result if the calcium oxide came into contact with the skin. The sachets have a short life and must be kept in an air-tight container, as they absorb moisture from the air.

Experiment 15.4 To demonstrate heat perming.
Prepare a heat perm lotion by dissolving 10 g of sodium bisulphite in 100 ml of water and adding 1 ml of 0·880 ammonium hydroxide. Soak a test curler of cut hair in the lotion for a few minutes, and then steam it in a conical flask as shown in Fig. 15.4 for 20 minutes. Wash the curler in warm water and dry it.

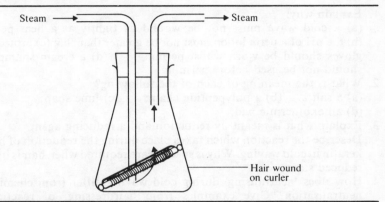

Fig. 15.4 Demonstration of heat perming

Hair straightening

The straightening of over-curly hair may be carried out by the same chemical process as the waving or curling of straight hair. The hair is treated with 10 per cent ammonium thioglycollate in a thick emulsion and wound on large rollers or combed straight until the curls are relaxed or softened by the breakage of cystine linkages. Breakage of the hair itself may result if combing is continued when the hair is in its weakened reduced state. After rinsing away the reducing agent, hydrogen peroxide is used to oxidise the cysteine and re-form cystine so setting the hair in its new straight shape.

On very tightly curled hair, a cream containing 5 per cent of sodium hydroxide may be used as the straightener. The cream is caustic with a pH of about 12 so the scalp must be protected by applying petroleum jelly. A back-wash basin should be used when washing the solution off the hair, to avoid damage to the client's eyes and skin. An acid rinse to neutralise any alkali left on the hair would then be beneficial.

Less damaging products with a pH of 8 are now available. They contain reducing agents such as sodium bisulphite or ammonium bisulphite with sodium lauryl sulphate as a wetting agent. After application of the lotion, heat from a hair dryer is required for about 15 minutes to speed the breaking of the disulphide bonds. The hair is then combed straight for 15 minutes. Oxidation by hydrogen peroxide is carried out after rinsing off the reducing agent. Disulphide bonds in the cystine linkages are formed in new positions along the polypeptide chains thus permanently setting the hair in the straightened state.

Questions

1. Explain why:
   (a) a cold wave must not be wound as tightly as a heat perm;
   (b) the pH of a perm lotion must not be greater than 9·5; (c) protective gloves should be worn whilst perming;   (d) a cream shampoo should not be used before perming.
2. What is the meaning of each of the following?
   (a) a salt;   (b) a polypeptide chain;   (c) lime soap;
   (d) an exothermic pad.
3. Explain what is meant by reduction and a reducing agent.
   Describe the reaction which takes place during the reduction of hair keratin in cold waving. Why is special care required when hair is in its reduced state?
4. How does 'neutralising' during cold waving differ from chemical neutralisation? Give examples from hairdressing, of reactions involving chemical neutralisation.
5. What is the effect on hair of   (a) dilute sodium hydroxide solution and   (b) concentrated sodium hydroxide solution?
   For what purposes may sodium hydroxide be used in a salon?

Part 4
Diseases, safety and first aid

Chapter 16

Disease in the salon

During the course of their work hairdressers will inevitably encounter various infections, non-infectious conditions and infestations of the hair and scalp. They should be able to recognise common diseases and conditions, so that they can judge the advisability of carrying out various hairdressing processes. They must also protect themselves and their clients from infection. The hairdresser is not expected to treat these conditions, but must use tact and understanding in referring the client to a doctor when necessary.

Infection and its effect on the body

An infectious disease is one which can be passed from one person to another. Infection itself is caused by the presence of micro-organisms which may be classified as *fungi*, *bacteria* and *viruses*. Fungi tend to grow on the outside of the body, as for example the ringworm fungus of the scalp, and to take nourishment from the skin. Although there are many differences between them, disease-causing bacteria and viruses are commonly known as *'germs'*. They cause disease when they enter body tissues, multiply and either destroy body cells by breaking them up or by producing poisons (toxins) which damage the cells. If they enter the body through the mouth they may affect the digestive system, causing diseases such as food poisoning, dysentery and typhoid fever. The air breathed in may carry germs which attack the lining of the nose, throat or lungs causing colds, sore throats, influenza and other diseases of the respiratory tract. Entry of germs through breaks in the skin leads to impetigo and boils, and often enables germs to pass into the blood stream. Germs may also multiply in the hair follicles giving rise to boils, folliculitis (infection of the follicles) and to the formation of pustules in cases of acne.

The body defends itself in several ways from attacks by germs. Many germs are destroyed by white blood cells (phagocytes) which surround and digest bacteria. Others are killed by chemical antibodies produced in the body and circulated in the blood stream. These either attack the germs themselves or provide antitoxins to counteract the poisons produced by some bacteria. The blood supply to an infected area is always increased so that the area looks red or inflamed. The body temperature may also be raised, producing fever. This speeds up the chemical changes required for the attack on the invading germs.

Fungi and fungal diseases

Fungi are a group of plants which contain no green colouring matter (chlorophyll) and are unable, therefore, to make their food from the carbon dioxide of the air and water from the soil. They take nourishment from the material or living organism on which they grow. Fungi include yeasts and moulds.

In man, fungi cause ringworm of the skin and scalp, and athlete's foot (see Fig. 16.1). The fungus consists of a mass of long thread-like cells called a *mycelium*. The threads grow into the epidermis including the hair shafts, and secrete a juice which digests keratin for the nutrition of the fungus.

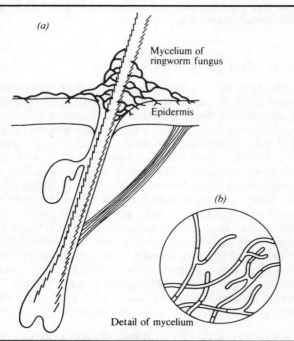

(a)

Mycelium of
ringworm fungus

Epidermis

(b)

Detail of mycelium

Fig. 16.1 (*a*) Hair follicle showing ringworm fungus
(*b*) Detail of mycelium

Ringworm of the scalp appears as a round patch of greyish scaly skin with short stubbly broken-off hairs. The hair shafts become weak and break due to digestion of the hair keratin by the fungus. Some inflammation of the patch may occur. Ringworm is more frequently seen in children than in adults. It is spread by direct contact with an infected head, or may be spread by broken off infected hairs in brushes, on towels, or in hats. The disease used to be cured by complete removal of the hair or epilation by X-rays. The drug griseofulvin is now given orally. It circulates in the blood, and is taken up by any newly formed keratin of the skin or hair which is then protected from infection. The old infected hair can be cut off as it grows.

Favus or honeycomb ringworm is a rare form of scalp ringworm. It is characterised by yellow crusts and a mousey smell and may lead to permanent bald patches.

Ringworm of the body, nails and beard are also caused by different types of fungus.

Athlete's foot (ringworm of the foot) is due to a fungus which grows between the toes, especially between the fourth and little toes. It appears as a wet spongy white patch, which later becomes dry and scaly. After a resting period it may break out again. If left untreated it may affect other toes and the ball of the foot. It is usually spread from person to person in places such as swimming baths or changing rooms where people walk barefoot.

Bacteria and bacterial diseases

Bacteria are present almost everywhere around us; in the air, soil and in water and on most surfaces including the surface of the skin. Bacteria which cause disease are called *pathogens*, though many bacteria are harmless or non-pathogenic, as for example those used to make yoghurt.

Bacteria are too small to be seen individually by the naked eye, but may be seen through a microscope. Each bacterium consists of a single cell which is a complete unit of life. Food and oxygen enter through the cell membrane and waste products leave the cell. If conditions are favourable, bacteria reproduce themselves by splitting into two. This may take place every twenty minutes. Bacteria can be cultured or grown into a *colony* which is easily seen by the naked eye, and can be used to identify the type of bacteria.

Conditions required for the growth of bacteria

In order to multiply, bacteria require:
1. A supply of food.
2. A supply of moisture. Dryness can prevent growth. Complete lack of moisture can kill bacteria.
3. A suitable temperature. Low temperatures, as in refrigeration, prevent growth but do not kill bacteria. Most bacteria except spore-bearing types are killed by a temperature of 70°C.
4. A supply of oxygen (usually).
5. Darkness. Bacteria are destroyed by the ultra-violet rays in sunlight.
6. Slightly alkaline conditions (pH 7–8).

7. Freedom from certain chemicals. Bacteria are killed if exposed to chemical disinfectants of sufficient concentration and for sufficient time. Chemical antiseptics inhibit the growth of bacteria but do not necessarily kill them.

The classification of bacteria

Bacteria may be classified by shape as shown in Table 16.1. Cocci cannot move by themselves but some bacilli have thread-like projections called *flagella*, which propel them through liquids. Spirochaetes move with a rotary action.

Some bacteria develop *spores* with a tough coat. They can survive adverse conditions and become active again when conditions improve.

Table 16.1 Classification of bacteria

Type of bacteria		Diseases
1. Cocci (spherical)		
(a) streptococci form chains		Impetigo, sore throats
(b) staphylococci form bunches		Boils
(c) diplococci form pairs		Pneumonia
2. Bacilli (rod shaped)		Diphtheria, typhoid
3. Spirochaetes (spiral shaped)		Venereal diseases

Experiment 16.1　The growth of bacteria on agar plates
Obtain a series of sterile petri dishes containing nutrient agar. Using swabs of sterile cotton wool, wipe various salon tools and transfer any bacteria to an agar plate by gently pressing the cotton wool on the surface of the agar. Use a different plate for each of the following:

1 A comb which has been standing in a bowl of antiseptic.
2. A brush after brushing a head.
3. The same brush after being placed in a salon sterilising cabinet for 15 minutes.

Also prepare plates as follows:
4. Place a scalp hair on the agar.
5. Touch the plate with three separate finger-tips.
6. Repeat (5) after washing the hands.
7. Expose a plate to the air for ten minutes.

Place the dishes in an incubator at 37°C for a few days, then examine the colonies preferably without removing the lids in case pathogens are present.

Bacterial infection in the salon

Bacterial infections which may be encountered in a salon include impetigo, boils, acne and sore throats.

Impetigo is caused by streptococci which enter breaks in the skin. The mouth area in children is often affected. Bacteria invade the epidermis causing small blisters filled with clear liquid which later becomes thick and forms a yellow crust. The infection spreads easily over the surface of the skin and is readily passed from person to person by infected towels or by touching the infected area. Impetigo may follow the breaking of the skin by lice or itch mites. Medical attention is required.

Boils are due to the multiplication of staphylococci in the tissue of a hair follicle. They often occur on the back of the neck just below the hair line, possibly due to a scratch with a dirty comb or to the rubbing of a dirty collar. The blood supply to the area is increased, making a hot inflamed lump. The bacteria are attacked by white blood cells which invade the area. Some bacteria and white cells are destroyed and form pus, which is later released from the 'head' of the boil. Since live bacteria are also present in pus, any dressings or materials used to clean the skin after the boil has burst, should be burned and the hands washed immediately.

Acne is basically caused by the blockage of the mouth of a hair follicle with a plug of keratin and sebum. Oxidation of the plug makes it black, forming a blackhead or comedo. Staphylococci, which are always present in follicles, may begin to multiply in the sebum plug and cause the formation of a pustule. The condition often affects adolescents due to an increased secretion of sebum at that period. Frequent washing helps to remove sebum but acne can be very disfiguring, and if at all severe requires medical attention. The plug causing the blackhead is not infectious, but if pus develops the condition must be treated as an infection.

Viruses and virus diseases

Viruses are smaller than bacteria and can only be seen under an electron microscope. They cannot be cultured like bacteria as they will only multiply inside a living cell. Viruses destroy the cells in which they live. For example, poliomyelitis viruses destroy nerve cells causing paralysis of the limbs. Virus diseases are, in general, more difficult to control than bacterial diseases. Viruses cause colds, influenza, measles, simple herpes, warts, AIDS and hepatitis B.

Many of these diseases are carried in drops of moisture from the nose and throat of an infected person during speaking, coughing or sneezing. The symptoms often start as **a cold** with soreness at the back of the nose and throat, followed by a watery discharge from the nose. In **measles** this is followed by a rash on the body. In **influenza** there is a sharp rise of temperature and aching of the limbs, and the patient should be confined to bed.

Simple herpes or cold sore is a recurring blister on the lip, which later forms a crust oozing moisture. The spot usually clears within a few days, but tends to recur when the person is over-tired or has a cold. The virus infection of the epidermis which causes this condition is usually contracted in childhood. The virus remains in the skin but the symptoms only occur in times of stress.

Warts on the hands of hairdressers are unsightly as well as being contagious and clients may object to them. Although warts tend to disappear eventually without treatment, it is advisable to have them removed by a doctor.

AIDS is caused by a virus known as HIV (Human Immunodeficiency Virus). This attacks blood cells which normally produce antibodies to fight infection. The AIDS patient may die from any infection which the body is unable to overcome due to lack of suitable antibodies. It may be transmitted during sexual intercourse or by injection into the blood stream using infected needles (often by drug addicts). In a salon, the risk of passing the virus from person to person is slight, but a small amount of blood or serum from an infected person may enter the blood of a healthy person if a tool such as scissors breaks the skin of both people. There is no risk of AIDS if the skin remains intact. Though the life of the virus on inanimate objects is short, sterilisation of tools is essential to safeguard clients.

Hepatitis B is a disease of the liver and may be transmitted through breaks in the skin in the same way as AIDS.

Infestation by animal parasites

A parasite is a living creature which obtains its food supply by living on or in the body of another living organism. Parasites living inside the body of their host are called *endoparasites* and include various worms which inhabit the digestive tract. Those living on the outside of the body are *ectoparasites* and it is with these that the hairdresser is most concerned. The presence of small animal parasites on the body is known as an *infestation*. This is not an infection in itself but often leads to *secondary infection* such as impetigo or boils, if bacteria enter breaks in the skin caused either by the bites of the parasite or scratching by the host.

Common parasites include:

1. The head louse (pediculus capitis)
Infestation by lice is known as *pediculosis*. Head lice (see Fig. 16.2) are usually found in the occipital region of the scalp but may spread to the parietal region. The adult female is about 2–3 millimetres in length and 1 millimetre in breadth and the male is slightly smaller. The louse has six legs, each ending in a claw with which it clings to the hair shafts. It feeds by piercing the skin of the host and sucking the blood. The female lays about 300 eggs, called *nits* (see Fig. 16.3), in a life of 4–5 weeks. The nits are white and shiny, and are oval in shape. A gummy cement firmly attaches them to the hair, usually close to the scalp. The eggs take about a week to hatch, and the young a week to mature. They are then capable of reproducing themselves.

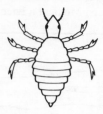

Fig. 16.2 Head louse

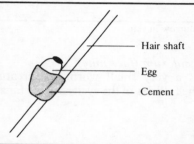

Hair shaft

Egg

Cement

Fig. 16.3 Nit attached to a hair

A lotion containing either 0·5 per cent *malathion* or 0·5 per cent *carbaryl* as an insecticide will kill both lice and nits after about two hours contact time when applied to dry hair. Nits are most resistant. Malathion clings electrostatically to hair and if the lotion is left on the hair for twelve hours before shampooing, complete bonding results and re-infestation will be prevented. Any dead nits or lice remaining on the hair after shampooing may be removed with a fine toothed comb. The hair should be allowed to dry naturally without the use of a hair dryer since both types of insecticide are destroyed by heat. The lotions must be stored in a cool place at below 25°C. Contact of the lotion with the eyes should be avoided. Although they may contain the same insecticides, lotions are more effective than shampoos since they have a longer contact time with the hair.

Lice are easily passed from person to person by direct contact or by the use of infested objects such as brushes or gowns.

2. The itch mite

The itch mite is a small eight-legged parasite which burrows into the epidermis causing a condition known as *scabies*. The burrows can be seen as dark lines about ten millimetres long under the skin, often between the fingers or in the folds at the front of the wrists. Intense irritation is caused, and small lumps and blisters may appear. The female, which is about 0·3 millimetres long and 0·2 millimetres wide, lays 40–50 eggs in the burrow (see Fig. 16.4). The eggs hatch in 4–8 days, and the young leave the burrow to live in the hair follicles. Impetigo or boils may result from secondary infection of breaks in the skin. Scabies is easily passed from person to person by direct contact, or through infested objects such as sheets. Medical advice is required.

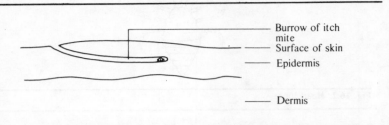

Fig. 16.4 Itch mite burrow in skin

3. *Demodex folliculorum (face mite)*

The face mite is a very small worm-like creature which inhabits blackheads and the follicles of the eyelashes. As far as is known, the face mite is harmless.

Non-infectious conditions

Psoriasis

Psoriasis is caused by an abnormal formation of skin keratin. Thick patches of silvery scales are to be found on the scalp, and often on the knees and elbows. There may be thimble-pitting of the surface of the nails. Under the scales, the skin may be red and small bleeding points may occur if the scales are removed. The patches may clear on medical treatment, but often recur, particularly in times of stress. Psoriasis often runs in families and is non infectious. Normal hairdressing treatments may be carried out.

Alopecia

Alopecia is a general term meaning *baldness*. *Alopecia totalis* refers to the complete loss of all scalp hair, and *alopecia universalis* to the complete loss of hair from all parts of the body. In *alopecia areata*, baldness occurs in small patches which often follow the line of a nerve. The areas are completely bald, with no broken-off hairs such as those found in ringworm (see Fig. 16.5). Alopecia areata is thought to be of nervous origin and the hair usually regrows after a period. *Traction alopecia* may be caused by constantly drawing the hair back tightly as in a pony tail which causes the hair line to recede at the front margin. Similar hair loss may result from over-vigorous brushing, the use of too tight curlers or tight plaiting (see Fig. 16.6).

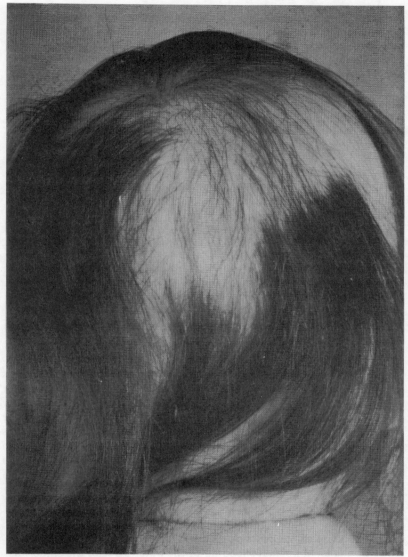

Fig. 16.5 Alopecia areata

Dermatitis

Dermatitis is an inflammation of the skin caused by contact with an irritant substance. A *primary irritant* causes inflammation on its first contact with the skin. A *secondary irritant* or *sensitiser* causes inflammation in certain people who have already had previous contact with the

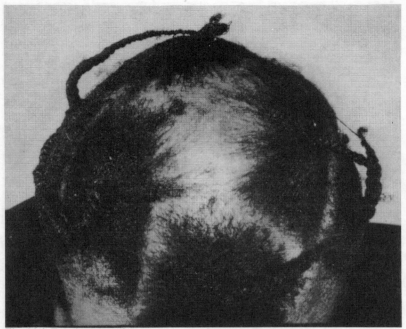

Fig. 16.6 Traction alopecia

substance without ill effect. They are then said to be allergic to the substance and further contact should be avoided. The symptoms of dermatitis appear a few hours after contact with the substance and may persist for some days. They may be mild with slight reddening of the skin or may result in serious swelling of the tissues or blistering and cracking of the skin. The hairdressing products most commonly causing contact dermatitis include oxidation dyes, ammonium thioglycollate, lanolin and sodium lauryl sulphate. As a precaution against dermatitis clients should be given a skin test before the application of oxidation dyes, and hairdressers should wear protective gloves when applying perm lotion or tints.

Dandruff (pityriasis)

Dandruff consists of patches of small dry scales on the scalp. The condition is an abnormal shedding of the outer layer of the epidermis. In severe cases, grey or white scales are constantly falling from the scalp and this may be accompanied by itching. The accumulation of scales on the scalp provides a good breeding ground for bacteria and yeast cells which are always associated with dandruff. Medicated shampoos are beneficial and keep infection to a minimum, but in severe cases shampoos containing selenium sulphide or zinc pyrithione are required to remove the keratin scales. They may also be removed by the use of *keratolytic* (keratin splitting) ointments containing salicylic acid.

Simple dandruff may be complicated by increased activity of the sebaceous glands. Oily accumulations of scales develop and the condition is known as *seborrhoea*.

Eye infections such as *blepharitis* (inflammation and thickening of the eyelids) and *conjunctivitis* (inflammation of the mucous membrane covering the eye ball) may be caused by irritation and bacterial infection due to dandruff falling into the eyes.

Defects of the hair shaft

The hair shaft may be damaged mechanically by severe back combing or back brushing, by the use of spiked rollers or excessively tight rollers. Chemical damage to the hair may result from the use of any very alkaline products (pH greater than 9·5) or by too strong perm lotion or bleaches. Defects of the hair shaft may be due to changes in the follicle itself which affect hair growth.

The defects include:

1. Fragilitas crinium
If the hair becomes very dry and brittle, it often splits either at the ends or at various points along the shaft. Split ends may be made to cling together slightly by use of protein hydrolysate conditioners. This is an electrostatic effect and not a permanent repair. Split ends should be cut off. Hot oil treatments using vegetable oils such as olive or almond oil are beneficial, or cetrimide-based conditioning rinses may be used. The condition is caused by either mechanical or chemical damage.

2. Trichorrhexis nodosa
In this condition nodes or small split swellings appear on the hair shaft (see Fig. 16.7). The hair often breaks off at the nodes. The condition is due to mechanical or chemical damage.

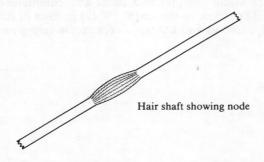

Hair shaft showing node

Fig. 16.7 Trichorrhexis nodosa

3. Monilethrix

This is a rare hereditary condition in which the thickness of the hair shaft varies along its length, leading to a beaded hair shaft. It is due to rhythmic changes in hair growth in the follicle (see Fig. 16.8).

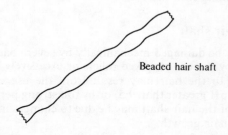

Beaded hair shaft

Fig. 16.8 Monilethrix

Questions

1. If a bacterium divides into two every 20 minutes under favourable conditions, how many bacteria would be produced in 8 hours from a single bacterium?

2. Explain the following terms:
   (a) infectious;   (b) contagious;   (c) pathogenic;   (d) toxic.

3. Explain how you would proceed if:
   (a) a client had dry hair with split ends;   (b) a client had severe dandruff;   (c) your client were infested by lice.

4. What steps should a hairdresser take to keep her hands in good condition and avoid dermatitis?

5. What advice would you give to a client who complained of:
   (a) small bald patches on the scalp?   (b) patches of silvery scales on the scalp, elbows and knees?   (c) excessively greasy hair?

Chapter 17

Prevention of the spread of infection

Hairdressers have a duty to their clients to prevent the spread of infection in the salon as far as possible. The close contact between hairdresser and client, the ease with which infections can be passed on by infected tools, and the warm, moist conditions of the salon provide ideal conditions for the spread of infection unless special attention is given to personal and salon hygiene, the sterilisation of tools, and salon ventilation.

How infection is spread

In a salon, infection may be spread from one person to another by the following methods:

1. Direct contact with the infected person:
(a) by droplet infection through inhaling air-borne droplets coming from the nose or mouth of an infected person whilst coughing, sneezing, or speaking. Colds, influenza and measles may be spread in this way.
(b) by touching an infected area of a person's body. Ringworm, impetigo and boils may spread by touch.

2. Indirect contact through use of an infected tool or contact with infected hair or towel. This involves cross-infection which is the passing of infection from a person to an object and the subsequent transfer of that infection from the object to a second person. The two people involved may never actually meet and could have entered the salon on completely different occasions. Ringworm fungus may be transmitted via hair brushes, and impetigo through infected towels. More seriously, AIDS (Acquired Immune Deficiency Syndrome) and hepatitis B could possibly be transmitted if a tool, contaminated by infected blood or serum from one client (or hairdresser), pierced the skin of a second client (or hairdresser). There is no danger of infection from AIDS or hepatitis if the skin remains intact. It is impossible to know if any particular client or hairdresser is carrying either of these infections, but good salon hygiene and sterilisation of tools will eliminate the risk of transmission of infection.

The control of infection

Infection by direct contact can be minimised by good salon hygiene and common sense. Staff with heavy colds should stay at home. Clients with colds increase the amount of air-borne infection but the effect may be reduced by improving the ventilation. If clients have obvious skin infections such as ringworm, it must be tactfully suggested that they consult a doctor and no hairdressing service should be given. Where the condition is unnoticed until work has begun, complete the service as briefly as possible. Tools which have been in contact with the client must be sterilised by autoclave if possible and other equipment disinfected. Clients with minor skin conditions such as boils or eczema may be treated normally, using disposable towels and gowns and using tools which can be autoclaved before use on another client. Affected areas of the skin should not be touched.

To avoid transfer of germs by indirect contact, each hairdresser should have two sets of tools to allow time for autoclaving, if necessary, between clients. Good salon hygiene and the sterilisation of tools will minimise the transmission of infection. During use, combs and other tools should be placed on a clean paper towel on the dressing table, and never in an overall pocket. Each client requires clean towels. Drying used towels without first washing them is unhygienic, as germs will multiply in the warmth during drying. In machine laundering towels, gowns and nets, use of the hottest wash possible, according to the type of fabric, will reduce infection.

Pathogens may be transferred from the hairdresser's hands to other objects if strict personal hygiene is not observed. The hands should always be washed after using the lavatory, after blowing the nose, and before and after attending to a client.

The treatment of tools

The incidence of AIDS and hepatitis B has led to greater concern about methods of sterilisation of salon tools. **Sterilisation** means the complete destruction of all living organisms on an object. This can rarely be achieved in a salon except by the use of an autoclave, or by dry heat using high temperatures for an adequate period of time.

Methods of sterilisation

1. By moist heat
Boiling water or steam treatment will not sterilise tools unless

accompanied by increased pressure as in the *autoclave*. This works on the same principle as a domestic pressure cooker (see Fig. 17.1). If water vapour is not allowed to escape from the container in which water is being heated, the pressure on the surface of the water is increased. This makes it more difficult for the molecules to leave the water until they are given more energy by raising the temperature. Thus increasing the pressure raises the boiling point of water. At normal atmospheric pressure water boils at 100°C but on doubling the pressure the boiling point rises to about 120°C. Autoclaving is suitable for metal tools, glass, and rubber objects as well as some plastics. Electrically controlled automatic autoclaves are available and should be used according to the manufacturer's instructions. The process of sterilisation takes about fifteen minutes at a temperature of around 120°C.

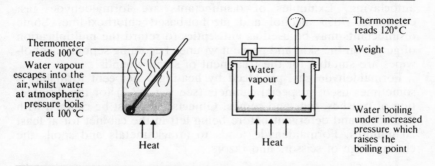

Fig. 17.1 Increasing the pressure raises the boiling point

Immediate autoclaving is essential for tools such as scissors and crochet hooks if they have pierced the skin of either a client or a hairdresser. This avoids the possible transfer of infected blood to the blood stream of a second person. Such contaminated tools must not be used again before sterilisation. They should be placed on a paper towel until treated by autoclaving and the towel immediately burned or enclosed in a plastic bag and sealed before disposal. Crochet hooks, and the removable blades of clippers should be autoclaved regularly. Scissors may be blunted during autoclaving and, unless they have penetrated the skin, are normally washed in detergent and water then dried, or wiped with a prepared alcohol-wipe and left to dry.

Boiling in water at 100°C for 15 minutes before washing is a suitable means of reducing infection on towels.

2. Dry heat
Glass bead sterilisers using dry heat may be used instead of an autoclave but need 30 minutes to heat before sterilisation can

commence, will generally take only one long instrument at once, are unsuitable for such items as clipper blades and, since they work at higher temperatures, tend to blunt or damage tools more. They should be used according to manufacturer's instructions since the time required for sterilisation depends on the temperature attained.

Naked flames may be used to treat small metal tools but blunting may occur and the method has little practical value in hairdressing.

Burning destroys pathogens and salon rubbish such as cut hair and infected tissues may be disposed of by this method.

The use of disinfectants

Chemical disinfectants are substances which will kill germs if used strong enough and long enough. They are unsuitable for sterilising tools but may be used to reduce the risk of infection from equipment such as brushes, rollers and combs which are unsuitable for autoclaving. Examples of disinfectants are formaldehyde gas, cetrimide, 70% alcohol and alcohol-based chlorhexidine. Some disinfectants may be used as **antiseptics** to retard the multiplication of germs on the skin and prevent wounds becoming septic. Alcohol-wipes are suitable for the treatment of small wounds.

Formaldehyde gas, produced by heating 5 per cent formalin, is sometimes used in special cabinets (see Fig. 17.2) for the disinfection of brushes, nets and combs. Objects must first be cleaned with hot water and detergent before being left in the cabinet for at least 20 minutes. Formaldehyde tends to attack metals and spoils the cutting edge of scissors and razors.

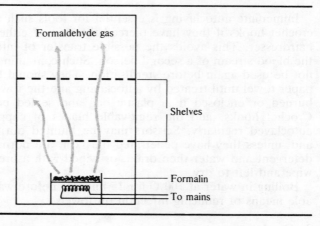

Fig. 17.2 Formaldehyde cabinet

Liquid disinfectants such as cetrimide or chloroxylenol are some-times used as a bath for combs. Unless care is taken to maintain the correct concentration and to replace the disinfectant regularly the method has little value. Alternatively combs could be washed with hot water and detergent after use on a client and wiped with a prepared alcohol-wipe. The blades of electrical clippers should also be regularly treated with an alcohol-wipe.

The use of ultra-violet radiation

Ultra-violet cabinets are used in many salons and, since the rays have only disinfectant properties, are useful for storing tools previously sterilised by autoclave. The rays are produced by a mercury vapour lamp at the top of the cabinet and travel in straight lines so that objects must be turned frequently to expose all surfaces to the rays. Since the rays are damaging to the eyes and skin, the lamp normally switches off when the cabinet door is opened.

Salon hygiene

Along with personal hygiene and the cleanliness of tools, the clean-liness of the salon itself and its furnishings is important in preventing the spread of infection. Surfaces of dressing tables, basins, walls, floors, and chairs must be cleaned regularly by washing with hot water and detergent. Smooth surfaces are preferable since they do not readily hold dust and dirt. Dust may be inorganic such as ash from cigarettes and particles of grit from roads, or organic such as flakes of dead skin, small pieces of hair and fluff from clothing and towels. Dust mixed with moisture or grease forms dirt. This is best removed by use of a detergent and hot water, with an abrasive powder to break up the dirt if necessary.

Questions

1. How would you treat each of the following to minimise the risk of infection: (a) combs; (b) scissors; (c) towels; (d) neck shears; (e) hairbrushes.
2. Explain the difference between:
   (a) disinfectants and antiseptics; (b) infection spread by direct and indirect contact; (c) sterilisation and disinfection.

3. Describe the action you would take in each of the following cases:
   (a) you have accidentally cut the lobe of a client's ear;
   (b) you suspect ringworm on a client's scalp;
   (c) your client is suffering from a boil on the neck.
4. List the materials most suitable for each of the following:
   (a) the surface of a dressing table;   (b) salon floors;
   (c) salon walls;   (d) the upholstry of chairs.
   Give reasons for your choice
5. Explain how the following may be passed from person to person:
   (a) head lice: (b) colds;   (c) impetigo;   (d) athlete's foot.

Chapter 18

Personal hygiene and posture

Hairdressers often work in conditions which are far from ideal. They tend to stand for long hours, and are thus subject to foot troubles which may lead to bad posture and fatigue. Unless the ventilation is good, the salon may become too hot and humid, making the hairdresser perspire freely and become uncomfortable and irritable. Many of the substances used are damaging to the skin, the hands particularly being at risk, and special care must be taken to keep them in good condition. Clients notice the state of the hairdresser's skin, nails, hair and clothing. It is essential not only to have a clean and tidy salon, but also that hairdressers themselves present a well-groomed appearance and avoid giving offence to clients by perspiration or breath odours.

Care of the skin

There are two types of sweat glands in the skin:

1. The eccrine or sudoriferous glands (see Fig. 18.1)
These are found practically all over the surface of the body and secrete perspiration consisting of salt (2 per cent) and water (98 per cent) with traces of waste products such as urea and lactic acid.

In temperate climates, about 1 litre of eccrine sweat is secreted per day without the skin becoming wet. This is known as *insensible perspiration*. The secretion of perspiration is increased by heat and nervous tension.

2. The apocrine glands
These are located in the arm-pits and produce perspiration with a more fatty content. This type of perspiration is readily attacked by bacteria, which break it down to substances with an unpleasant odour.

A daily bath is necessary to remove both types of sweat, and also to remove dead skin, dirt, bacteria, make-up and excess sebum. Underclothing which absorbs perspiration from the skin should be changed daily.

Underarm sweating may be reduced by the use of *anti-perspirants* containing astringents such as aluminium chlorhydrate. *Deodorants*, in the form of antiseptics such as cetrimide or hexachlorophane, are often

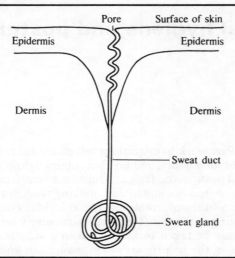

Fig. 18.1 Eccrine sweat gland

added to the anti-perspirant to prevent the multiplication of the bacteria which cause odour by breakdown of sweat.

The skin of the hands presents a special problem. A hairdresser's hands are often affected by the continual use of water and detergents during shampooing. Soapless shampoos in particular tend to remove the natural sebum from the skin surface. This oily layer normally keeps the skin supple by retaining moisture in the epidermis, enabling it to stretch and wrinkle without cracking. Lack of sebum enables additional water to enter the horny layer causing it to swell and later to become rough and chapped. Bacteria may enter the cracks in the skin causing infection. The loss of sebum may be reduced by applying barrier creams to the hands before starting work. Hand cream applied at night helps to replace the oily film on the skin.

Soapless detergents may also cause dermatitis. They should be rinsed thoroughly from the skin after use, particularly from the area between the fingers and under rings. Protective gloves should be worn when applying permanent dyes or perm lotion to avoid contact dermatitis.

Care of the nails

Nails (see Fig. 18.2) grow in a similar way to hair, by the division of cells in the germinating layer of the epidermis. Growth of nails takes place in the *nail matrix*. Both nails and hair consist mainly of the protein *keratin*.

The nail itself consists of four parts:
1. *The nail root*, which lies under the nail fold or cuticle.
2. *The lunula* or half moon.
3. *The nail plate* which forms the main body of the nail, and is

pink due to the blood vessels in the dermis below the nail.

4. *The projecting or free edge* of the nail which extends slightly beyond the end of the finger, and is detached from the skin.

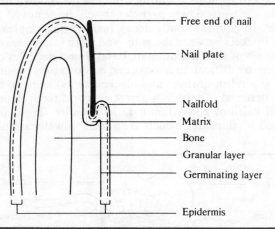

Free end of nail

Nail plate

Nailfold

Matrix

Bone

Granular layer

Germinating layer

Epidermis

Fig. 18.2 Section of the end of a finger

The under part of the nail rests on, and is firmly attached to, the nail bed of living epidermal cells. There is no granular layer under the nail plate, but it extends as far as the lunula. *The cuticle*, which is part of the horny layer of the epidermis, often extends on to the nail plate. Its function is to prevent infection reaching the nail matrix, and care should be taken not to damage the cuticle during manicuring. Infection may lead to an abcess, with possible damage to the growing nail.

Finger nails grow about 5 millimetres per month. Finger nails grow faster than thumb nails and also faster than toe nails. If a nail is lost by accident, complete regrowth takes about four months.

Nails should be kept clean and well manicured. Dirt under the nails provides a breeding ground for bacteria. Nails should be kept short so as not to scratch the client's scalp or catch in the client's hair. Strong detergents remove oil from nails, leaving them brittle. Nail enamel offers some protection against loss of oil.

Nail enamel consists of a plastic resin dissolved in a solvent such as ethyl acetate or amyl acetate. On the nail, the solvent evaporates and leaves a coating of coloured plastic. Glycerol is often added to nail enamel as a plasticiser, to keep the plastic soft and to prevent flaking.

Plastic resin + amyl acetate = nail enamel
  (solute)   (solvent)   (a solution)

Nail enamel can be removed by ethyl acetate or amyl acetate which redissolves the plastic film. Acetone is now rarely used as a solvent as it is considered to be too de-greasing to the skin and nail.

Care of the teeth and mouth

The enamel of teeth is the hardest substance in the human body, but it may be attacked by acids resulting from the breakdown of particles of food left on the teeth. These particles should be removed by brushing after meals, to prevent tooth decay (caries) and unpleasant breath (halitosis). Pockets between the gums and teeth sometimes occur due to the breakdown of the cementing material. Food particles collecting in these pockets are difficult to remove and halitosis may result. Vitamin C in the diet (found in oranges and blackcurrants) helps to build up the cementing material. The development of good teeth depends on the presence of calcium and vitamin D in the diet. Teeth may also be strengthened by fluorides, which are added to water supplies in some areas.

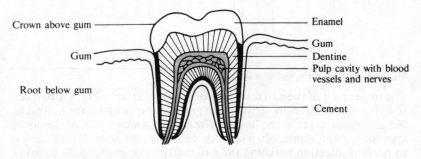

Fig. 18.3 Section of a tooth

Unpleasant breath may result from digestive troubles, and offence to clients can also be caused by smoking and by eating strong-smelling foods such as oranges, onions or garlic.

Care of the feet

Since hairdressers are standing most of the day, special care of the feet is required to avoid discomfort. A chiropodist should be consulted if any painful conditions arise.

The following foot conditions may need attention:

1. **Corns** are a thickening of the epidermis due to pressure by ill-fitting shoes.
2. **Ingrowing toenails** result from pressure on the nails. The condition may be eased by cutting the nails straight across or slightly concave.
3. **Bunions** (Hallux Valgus) are caused by incorrectly fitting shoes. The joint of the big toe becomes inflamed, causing pain and resulting in an unsightly-shaped foot.
4. **Flat feet** (Pes planus) and **fallen arches** (see Fig. 18.4) may be due to continual standing or may be inherited. The arches of the foot are

maintained by strong ligaments which are prevented from stretching by muscles in the legs. Strain and tiredness of these muscles can result in fallen arches. The condition may be treated by exercises or by an artificial support to the arches.

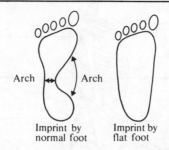

Arch   Arch

Imprint by   Imprint by
normal foot   flat foot

Fig. 18.4 Flat feet

5. **Athlete's foot** is a fungus infection resulting in soggy white patches between the toes. Medical attention is required.
6. **Plantar warts** are a form of ingrowing wart and can be very painful. A chiropodist should be consulted.

The above conditions can largely be avoided by attention to foot hygiene and the use of correct footwear. The feet should be washed frequently especially if they perspire freely. They should be dried well particularly between the toes, as warmth and moisture encourage the growth of fungus and bacteria. Dusting the feet with talcum powder will help to absorb sweat.

Shoes should grip at the heel and over the instep. The arch of the foot should be supported and there should be room for the toes to move easily inside the shoe. Very high heels tend to throw the body forward and this leads to bad posture. Claw toes may also result if the foot slips forward in the shoe due to high heels. A low or medium heel is usually more comfortable.

Posture

Bad posture can lead to both fatigue and lasting ill-health if strain is placed on muscles and ligaments, and if respiration and circulation are restricted by rounded shoulders causing compression of the chest. In addition, bad posture gives the client an impression of an unenthusiastic and careless worker. Clothes, too, do not look their best, and may hang unevenly, for they are made to fit a well balanced figure.

Posture is dependent on the skeleton, the ligaments which bind the bones together and the muscles which enable movement to take place. The skeleton is shown in Fig. 18.5. It consists of two parts, the *axial skeleton* comprising the skull, spine and rib-cage, and the *appendicular skeleton* which includes the bones of the limbs and also the pelvic (hip)

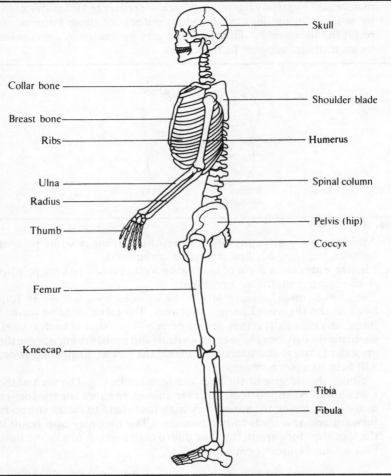

Fig. 18.5 The skeleton (side view showing only one arm and one leg)

and shoulder girdles. The skeleton has several important functions:

1. To support the body, giving it a rigid structure and enabling it to keep its shape.
2. To support internal organs; for example, the pelvis supports the abdominal organs.
3. To protect delicate organs. Thus the rib-cage protects the heart and lungs; the skull protects the brain.
4. To form a point of attachment for muscles enabling movement to take place.

The ligaments which strap the adjacent bones together are pliable and allow movement at the joints. In bad posture it is often the ligaments which suffer strain by being overstretched. The position of the ligaments can be seen in the *hinge joint* in Fig. 18.6. This type of joint, found at the elbow and knee, allows movement in one direction only. Other types of movable joint are the *ball and socket joint* found at the hips and shoulders, and the *plane or gliding joint* in which two flat surfaces move over each other, as in the wrist and the spine.

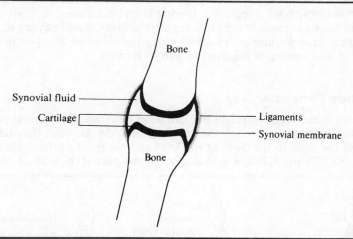

Fig. 18.6 Section through a hinge joint

Muscles are attached to bones by tendons which are non-elastic. When the muscles contract, the bones are pulled into a different position, as for example the movement of the forearm (see Fig. 18.7). Contraction of the biceps raises the forearm. Contraction of the triceps straightens the arm. These muscles which can be moved at will are called *voluntary muscles*. Muscles such as those in the heart and digestive tract

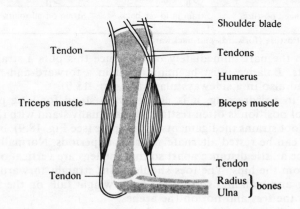

Fig. 18.7 Muscle action

are under the control of the brain, but not the will and are said to be *involuntary*.

Muscles are always in a state of slight contraction, ready to respond when movement is required. This condition is known as *muscle tone*. The contraction of muscle needs energy which is obtained chemically by the oxidation of the glucose brought to the muscle in the bloodstream, and stored there until required. During exercise, increase in heart rate and in breathing rate bring extra supplies of glucose and oxygen to the muscles. *Muscle fatigue* results if waste products accumulate in the muscle, and resting is required to allow recovery.

Posture during standing

Posture is correct if a straight line can be drawn from the mastoid bone just behind the ear, through the tip of the shoulder, through the middle line of the hips, to the front of the knee and the front of the ankle (see Fig. 18.8). *Posture fatigue* is caused when one part of the body is out of

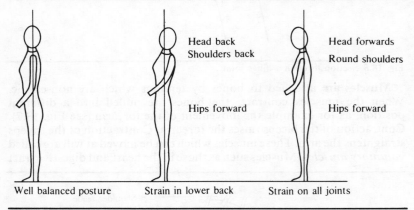

Well balanced posture   Strain in lower back   Strain on all joints

Fig. 18.8 Posture (forwards-and-backwards plane)

line with the part immediately below, since this puts a strain on the ligaments. Balance must be maintained in a forward-and-backward plane and also in a sideways plane (see Fig. 18.9).

If, as in hairdressing, it is necessary to stand for long periods, a change of position is often restful. To habitually stand with the weight on one foot strains the ligaments in the spine (see Fig. 18.9), but the leg muscles can be rested alternately for short periods. Normally the feet should be a little distance apart so that the legs are vertical or straight down from the hips. The toes should point straight forwards both in standing and walking, so that the body weight falls on the flat outer edges of the feet and not on the arches.

The shoulders should be level and point straight out to the sides. If the left shoulder is higher than the right, the lower spine bends to the left

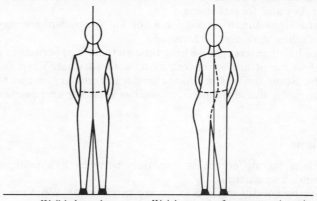

Well balanced posture   Weight on one foot curves the spine

Fig. 18.9 Posture (sideways plane)

and the ligaments on the left side of the spine become stretched. If the shoulders are brought forwards, the chest is compressed and the upper part of the back is rounded, so stretching the back muscles and ligaments. If the shoulders are pushed too far back, the natural curve of the back is flattened and this causes tension.

The head should be held straight up. If the chin drops, the line of vision is changed. If the chin is pushed outwards, the head tilts back causing strain in the neck and shoulder muscles. Holding the head on one side causes tension in the neck and shoulder muscles, as well as affecting vision since the eyes are on different levels.

Posture whilst sitting

In order that sitting should be restful, the back should be supported all the way down by sitting well back in the chair. There should be right angles at both hips and knees so that no tension occurs in the joints. The weight of the body should be supported by the pelvis and not by the bottom of the spine. Some of the weight of the thighs should be supported by the feet or there will be pressure on the blood vessels and nerves at the back of the thighs. Sitting with one leg over the other can result in similar pressure, and this may impair circulation causing the limb to 'go to sleep' or have 'pins and needles'.

Fatigue

Different forms of fatigue may be experienced by the hairdresser:
1. **Muscular fatigue** caused by prolonged working, which results in aching muscles and slowness of movement.
2. **Posture fatigue** due to strain on the muscles and ligaments by bad posture.

3. **Mental fatigue** due to prolonged mental activity results in frequent mistakes and forgetfulness.
4. **Heat fatigue** due to working in a hot, stuffy atmosphere may lead to headaches, dizziness or fainting.

Since hairdressers spend a long time on their feet, periods of rest with the feet raised are beneficial, along with adequate sleep and rest at night. Some form of outdoor exercise is necessary and will improve respiration and circulation, as well as relaxing nervous tension.

Questions

1. Explain the difference in function between ligaments, tendons, muscles and cartilage.
2. Working conditions in a salon are rarely ideal. What are the main drawbacks, and how can a hairdresser ensure that she retains her health and vitality?
3. What substances are removed from the skin during washing? Why is it desirable that they should be removed?
4. The following are basically solutions. List the solute and the solvent in each case.
   (a) formalin;   (b) nail enamel;   (c) hair lacquer;
   (d) vinegar rinse;   (e) perfume;   (f) hard water.
5. Explain what is meant by each of the following:
   (a) insensible perspiration;   (b) halitosis;   (c) muscle tone;
   (d) the nail matrix.

Chapter 19

Safety and First-aid

The Health and Safety at Work Act 1974 aims to secure the health, safety and welfare of all persons whilst at work. Under the Act, employers have a duty to their staff to carry out this aim by providing a safe and healthy environment. This includes the provision of safe and well-maintained equipment; safe methods of use and storage of dangerous materials; the cleanliness, heating, lighting and ventilation of premises; the provision of fire exits, fire fighting appliances and first-aid equipment; and adequate arrangements for the welfare of staff including washing and toilet facilities, and accommodation for outdoor clothing and overalls. The employer is also responsible for the training of staff in safety and health matters connected with their work and his duties are extended to ensure the safety and health of members of the public entering the salon. Employees, too, have a duty under the Act to take reasonable care for the health and safety of themselves and of persons who may be affected by their work.

The emphasis should be on the prevention of accidents but it is also essential to be able to deal efficiently with accidents if they do occur. All members of staff should know how to telephone for an ambulance or the Fire Service. They should understand the use of the salon fire extinguisher and know the position of the main stop-tap for water and the main switch for electricity. A knowledge of first-aid is essential. A torch should always be readily available for emergency use in case mains electricity supplies are unexpectedly cut off.

The prevention of accidents

Accidents involving falling may be minimised by ensuring that:
1. The salon is well lit, without any dark areas.
2. The floor has a non-slip surface and is kept free from spilled substances on which people may slip.
3. There are no trailing flexes to electrical appliances.
4. There are no dangerous projections on furniture and equipment.

Accidents resulting in electric shock may be avoided by:
1. The correct wiring and regular servicing of equipment including the replacement of frayed flexes and damaged plugs and switches.
2. Switching off at the mains before repairing fuses or switches.

3. Switching off the light switch before replacing lamps.
4. Disconnecting equipment for cleaning and examination for faults.
5. Never handling electrical equipment with wet hands or whilst standing on a wet floor.

Accidents with chemicals may usually be avoided by careful handling and by always following the manufacturer's instructions. In particular ensure that:
1. All containers are clearly labelled. Liquids should be poured from the side of the bottle opposite the label so that the label is not damaged by liquid running down the side of the bottle.
2. Chemicals are never placed in bottles commonly used for lemonade, squash, etc.
3. Once chemicals have been poured from storage bottles, any surplus is discarded and not poured back into the bottle.
4. Quantities are accurately measured and not merely guessed.
5. Chemicals are kept out of the way of children.
6. The stopper is replaced, and the bottle returned to its proper storage place immediately after use.
7. Chemicals do not run into client's eyes or on to the skin.
8. Protective gloves are always worn during perming or colouring.
9. The inhalation of lacquer is avoided.

Accidents to the client are avoidable by special care on the part of the hairdresser. Thus:
1. Cuts are most likely when cutting hair near the lobes of the ears and when cutting neck hairs.
2. The skin may be pierced when using hair pins or roller pins.
3. Burns may occur when using blow dryers, heat perm clips, exothermic pads and by placing metal clips next to the skin under a hairdryer.
4. Scalds may occur by using excessively hot water in shampooing, during the use of steamers, and when giving hot oil treatments.

Fire risks may be decreased by:
1. The careful use of flammable liquids such as petrol during wig cleaning, and alcohol-based products such as lacquer. These substances are always a potential fire risk, and should be stored in a metal bin in relatively small quantities. Hydrogen peroxide assists fire by giving off oxygen when heated and should not be stored near flammable substances.
2. The proper use of electrical equipment. Avoid overloading circuits, use the correct size of fuse for each appliance, and service equipment regularly to avoid faulty insulation and faulty appliances.
3. Never draping towels over convector heaters, dryers or storage heaters as this prevents the circulation of air, causing over-heating of the appliance.
4. Ensuring that cigarette ends are completely extinguished and that plenty of ashtrays are provided.

5. Avoiding the use of gloss paint on polystyrene ceiling tiles as this increases their flammability.
6. The careful use of gas appliances. These should be serviced regularly to ensure correct working. Radiant gas fires must be safely guarded and flammable materials kept at a distance. Escaping gas can explode if ignited and any suspected gas leak should be reported to the local Gas Board immediately. People should be asked to leave the salon, naked flames should be extinguished, the gas should be turned off at the main tap and doors and windows opened.

In the event of fire in the salon, the first consideration must be the safety of the occupants. A small fire may be tackled by a suitable fire extinguisher, but the clients should be asked to leave and the Fire Service called if the fire is not immediately extinguished. All windows and doors should be closed to reduce draughts which might fan the flames.

Fire fighting appliances must be available in every salon. Water must not be used on electrical fires or on burning oil. A compressed carbon dioxide type extinguisher (see Fig. 19.1) is suitable for salon use, but it should be tested quarterly by the Fire Service to maintain its efficiency. Sand is also useful on small fires. There should be regular fire drill and each member of staff should know how to deal with an emergency involving fire.

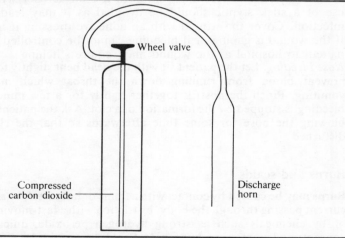

Fig. 19.1 Compressed carbon dioxide extinguisher

Wheel valve

Compressed carbon dioxide

Discharge horn

First aid

In cases of accident or illness in the salon, a hairdresser should be capable of rendering first aid. Regular clients may give information about their health during conversation and these comments should be mentally noted since it may be useful to know, in an emergency, that a client is a diabetic, has a heart condition or suffers from epilepsy. Such clients may also carry cards with instructions for treatment, and tablets or inhalants for emergency use. Most cases requiring attention in the salon will be minor accidents such as small cuts or slight burns. At the same time the hairdresser is responsible for the care and safety of clients and must deal with any emergency arising, however serious. It is important to stress the need for calling medical aid or an ambulance in good time if required, remembering also to pass on as much information as possible about the patient.

Bleeding

In all cases of bleeding, the aim of treatment is to prevent loss of blood and avoid infection of the wound.

Cuts and small punctured wounds. Minor cuts on the neck or lobe of the ear may be caused accidentally by scissors or razors, and small punctured wounds may result from the careless use of hair pins or roller pins. To check bleeding dab the wound with a prepared spirit swab and leave it to dry. Place the used swab in a plastic bag and seal before disposal. If bleeding continues use an aerosol styptic. The use of a stick styptic should be avoided as it may lead to cross infection. Cover the wound with an adhesive dressing if necessary. If the wound is gaping or if bleeding cannot be controlled, take the patient to hospital as the wound may require stitching.

Nose bleeding. Let the patient sit with the head bent slightly forward to prevent blood from running down the throat which may cause vomiting. Pinch the nostrils together tightly for a few minutes until bleeding is stopped by the formation of a clot. Ask the patient to avoid blowing the nose for some time afterwards so that the clot is not disturbed.

Burns and scalds

Burns may be caused by contact with a flame or hot metal, by an electric current passing through the body, by friction with a fast-moving object, or by chemicals such as strong hydrogen peroxide, quicklime, or concentrated ammonium hydroxide. **Scalds** have a similar effect on the skin to burns, but are caused by moist heat such as boiling water, steam or hot oil. Scalds caused by steam are often more severe than those caused by boiling water due to the latent heat given out as the steam condenses to water at 100°C. Burns and scalds result in intense pain with redness of the skin, blisters or in severe cases destruction of tissue. Burns due to electric current are often deep, but extensive burning of the skin surface is usually more serious.

Wash caustic chemicals off the skin immediately by flooding the area with cold water from a running tap, and remove any contaminated clothing as quickly as possible to prevent further burning. Treat other types of burns or scalds by running cold water gently over them from the tap or immersing them in cold water for 5–10 minutes to reduce the pain. If blisters occur, do not break them but cover them with a sterile dressing and bandage lightly. In severe cases cover the whole area including clothing, with a sterile dressing and remove the patient to hospital as soon as possible. At first the burnt skin and clothing will be sterile due to the effect of the heat, so avoid infection by covering it quickly and not touching the area or breathing over it. Reassure the patient, give cold drinks and keep the patient warm whilst awaiting transport to hospital.

Eye injuries

Small hairs or dust in the eyes.   Locate the foreign body by pulling down the lower eyelid. Remove the object with the corner of a clean handkerchief or a twist of cotton wool soaked in water. If it is thought to be under the upper lid, lift the upper lid over the lower one so that the lower lashes sweep the inner surface of the upper lid, or let the patient blink the eye under water using an eye bath. If unsuccessful, cover the eye with a sterile eye pad and take the patient to hospital.

Chemicals in the eye.   In the salon many hairdressing preparations such as perm lotions, shampoos, conditioners and bleaches may cause painful irritation of the eyeball if they accidentally enter the eye. Treat all cases by flushing the eye with large quantities of water poured gently from a jug, taking care that it does not enter the unaffected eye.

Fractures and sprains

A fracture (a broken bone) or a sprain may occasionally occur as a result of a fall in the salon.

Fractures.   These result in the loss of use, swelling and often distortion of the affected limb. The patient should not be moved but should be kept warm whilst awaiting the arrival of an ambulance. Do not give food or drink as the patient may require an anaesthetic for the setting of the bone.

Sprains.   These are due to the tearing of ligaments or other tissues round a joint, such as the ankle or wrist. Apply a crepe bandage and keep it wet with cold water to reduce any swelling. If the sprain is severe take the patient to hospital for an X-ray in case a bone is fractured.

Hysterical attacks

Nervous, highly excitable people are sometimes subject to hysterical attacks in times of emotional stress, but they usually like an audience and the attacks do not occur when the person is alone. The patient may laugh or cry uncontrollably, roll on the floor, or clutch at other people. Speak firmly without bullying and take the patient out of the salon to a quiet room. When sufficient control has been regained, keep the patient occupied.

Septic conditions

If a wound is not kept covered, bacteria of the staphylococcal type may enter the break in the skin, quickly multiply, and damage the surrounding tissue causing a septic condition. To counteract the infection, the blood supply to the wound increases and the area becomes red and inflamed. White blood cells leave the blood vessels and enter the tissues to attack the invading bacteria. Some bacteria and white cells are destroyed and together with dead tissue cells form a thick yellow discharge known as pus.

To treat a septic condition, bathe the area with hot water containing an antiseptic such as cetrimide, using cotton wool swabs. Cover the wound with an adhesive dressing to prevent the spread of infection and change the dressing frequently, bathing the wound with antiseptic each time. Since pus contains some live bacteria, burn all dressings and all materials used in cleansing the area and wash your hands immediately after attending to the wound.

Very small pieces of cut hair may sometimes enter a hairdresser's skin, particularly the soles of the feet, if cut hair falls into the shoes. This is a painful condition which quickly becomes septic if neglected. Remove the hair with tweezers using a magnifying glass if necessary, then bathe the area with antiseptic and cover with a sterile adhesive dressing.

Unconsciousness

There are many reasons for unconsciousness and, although it may be difficult for the hairdresser to detect the cause, the following general treatment should be carried out.

First make sure that the person can breathe freely, that the air passages are not blocked and that there is no restrictive clothing at the neck, waist or chest. Do not leave the patient, but ask someone to telephone for an ambulance immediately. If breathing normally, turn the patient onto one side with the upper arm at right angles to the body and the elbow bent, and the upper leg at right angles to the body with the knee bent. This positioning prevents the patient from rolling over on to the back and ensures that the air passages stay open and the person is not choked by the tongue or by swallowed saliva or vomit. This three-quarters prone position is sometimes known as the *recovery position*. Observe the patient constantly in case breathing begins to fail and artificial respiration is required. Do not attempt to give food or drink to an unconscious person to avoid choking. Keep the patient warm by covering with a blanket until the ambulance arrives, but do not give a hot-water bottle as this brings blood to the surface of the skin leaving less for vital internal organs.

Artificial respiration (mouth-to-mouth resuscitation) must be started at once as soon as breathing begins to fail, since lack of oxygen to the brain for more than a very few minutes would result in permanent brain damage. First ensure that the air passages are open by placing the casualty on his back, pressing the head backwards and the lower jaw upwards as shown in Figure 19.2. The patient's tongue is thus prevented from falling to the back of the throat so causing blockage of the air-way from the mouth and nose to the lungs.

After taking a deep breath surround the patient's mouth completely with your own lips, and at the same time pinch his nostrils together with your fingers. Blow into his lungs, stopping as soon as the chest has risen and then remove your mouth. Repeat the inflation of his lungs at your natural breathing rate until the patient starts breathing again or medical aid is obtained.

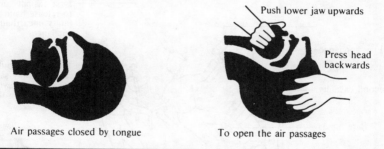

Push lower jaw upwards

Press head backwards

Air passages closed by tongue

To open the air passages

Fig. 19.2 Preparation for artificial respiration

The following conditions may all involve unconsciousness.

Concussion

This is caused by a blow to the head, possibly by striking the head on furniture when accidentally falling. The patient may be dazed or completely unconscious for a short time and may also suffer shock, so feeling sick and cold. Lay the patient down and cover with a blanket. Carry out the general treatment if unconscious and obtain medical aid.

Diabetic coma

Diabetes is caused by lack of insulin, a substance secreted by the pancreas which controls the level of sugar in the blood stream. A diabetic coma may result from either a **lack of insulin**, in which case the face would be flushed and the breathing deep with the breath smelling of acetone (nail enamel), or **an excess of insulin** when the skin would be pale and moist, and the breathing shallow but with no smell of acetone.

If still conscious, the patient may recover if given sugar lumps or a strongly sweetened drink. If the patient is unconscious apply the general rules for treatment and send for an ambulance.

Electric shock

Contact with faulty equipment which is not properly earthed, can lead to severe injury. The current causes violent contraction of muscle and the person may be unable to break contact with the live apparatus. The severity of the injury depends on the path the current takes as it passes to earth through the body. Breathing may stop due to paralysis of the muscles of respiration, and paralysis of the heart muscles may result in immediate death. Deep burns may also occur, but breathing should always be restored before burns are treated. On no account touch a person in contact with a live appliance without first insulating yourself (see Fig. 19.3).

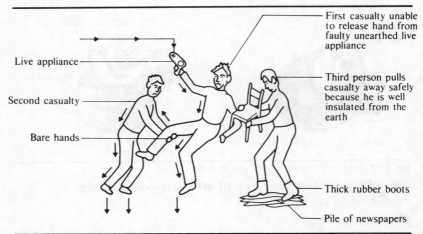

Live appliance

Second casualty

Bare hands

First casualty unable to release hand from faulty unearthed live appliance

Third person pulls casualty away safely because he is well insulated from the earth

Thick rubber boots

Pile of newspapers

Fig. 19.3 Electric shock

If possible switch off the current by removing the plug or by the main switch. The flex may be wrenched from the plug but must never be cut by scissors or a knife. If it is impossible to disconnect the current, insulate yourself with any dry insulating material. Stand on a pile of magazines or wear thick rubber-soled shoes and move the person away from the appliance with dry folded newspapers or a wooden chair protecting the hands with thick rubber gloves if possible.

If breathing has stopped apply artificial respiration which may need to be continued for some time. If you are alone do not stop to telephone for help until breathing is restored. Send for an ambulance as soon as possible.

Epilepsy

Epilepsy is a recurring condition often first appearing in young people. Fits vary in severity, the mildest involving only momentary loss of consciousness. In more severe cases, the patient may fall unconscious and after a few minutes the limbs may jerk violently due to uncontrollable contractions of the muscles. Do not restrain the movements, but prevent damage to the person by removing surrounding objects such as furniture. Place a knotted handkerchief in the patient's mouth to prevent the biting of the tongue. After the attack keep the patient warm and quiet to encourage sleep.

Fainting

Fainting is a common cause of unconsciousness and is due to an insufficient supply of blood to the brain. It may occur suddenly due to bad news or severe pain, or gradually due to fatigue or to sitting too long in a hot stuffy salon. If the person feels faint, loss of consciousness can often be avoided by lowering the head between the knees or using smelling salts. Increasing the supply of fresh air and unfastening tight clothing will also help. If fainting has actually taken place, lay the patient down with the head lower than the feet to increase the blood flow to the brain. Unconsciousness is usually brief and a drink of tea or sips of water may be given on recovery.

Heart attacks

Severe pains in the chest spreading to the arms, neck and the lower part of the face, are the symptoms leading to a heart attack. The patient may be short of breath and suffer serious shock resulting in unconsciousness. If still conscious support the person in a sitting position and loosen any tight clothing at the neck, chest or waist. Immediate hospital treatment is required. If breathing begins to fail commence artificial respiration at once. Test the pulse in the carotid artery in the neck alongside the larynx and if you are certain that there is no pulse and that the heart has therefore stopped beating, alternate breathing into the lungs with pressure over the heart. Place one hand on top of the other over the lower part of the breast bone and press the bone regularly at the rate of one press per second. Alternate one breath into the lungs with 5–7 presses over the heart until the ambulance arrives.

Poisoning

A person suspected of having swallowed any type of poison should be conveyed to hospital as quickly as possible and the bottle which held the poison should also be sent along for examination. If a *corrosive* substance such as strong ammonium hydroxide or household bleach has been swallowed, the lips and mouth will show white burns or blisters. In this case give large quantities of water or milk to drink to dilute the poison, and do not attempt to make the patient vomit or further damage to the oesophagus may result. If *non-corrosive* poisons such as overdoses of sleeping tablets or aspirin have been taken and the person is still conscious, try to cause vomiting by tickling the back of the throat with your fingers or a spoon. Do not let this delay despatch to hospital which may be by car if available. According to current medical opinion, attempts to cause vomiting by drinking an emetic solution of salt and water are dangerous and should not be practised. If unconscious, place the person in the recovery position so that choking is avoided if vomiting occurs. Keep the patient warm by covering with a blanket whilst waiting for the ambulance. If breathing shows signs of failing apply artificial respiration immediately.

Seizures

Seizures or strokes are most common in the middle-aged or elderly, and are caused either by bleeding from a burst blood vessel into the brain or by a blood clot blocking a blood vessel to the brain. The symptoms vary from loss of feeling or use of a limb, or slurred speech, to complete unconsciousness. Telephone for an ambulance immediately, and apply the general treatment for unconsciousness if necessary.

The first-aid box

The salon first aid box should contain the following equipment and should be restocked as soon as materials have been used:
- Prepared sterile dressings of various sizes including a sterile eye pad.
- Adhesive dressings of various sizes.
- Gauze bandages of various widths, a crepe bandage, a triangular bandage.
- A packet of sterilised cotton wool.
- Smelling salts, an eye bath, tweezers, scissors and safety pins.
- Antiseptic liquid and cream (cetrimide).
- A blanket should be stored near the first-aid box, together with a jug for rinsing chemicals from clients' eyes and a small basin and a cup.

Questions

1. Describe the action you would take to deal with a fire caused by a fault in a hairdryer.
2. Explain why:
   (a) hydrogen peroxide should not be stored near flammable substances;
   (b) water must not be used to extinguish electrical fires;
   (c) water must not be used to extinguish burning oil;
   (d) towels must not be draped over the air vents in hairdryers and storage heaters.
3. Explain why it is possible to resuscitate a person with the air being breathed out by the first aider.
4. What is meant by:
   (a) a corrosive poison?   (b) a septic cut?   (c) a sterile dressing?   (d) an emetic?
5. What is the difference between a burn and a scald?
   List the possible ways such injuries may occur in the salon.
   What action should be taken in giving first aid to these injuries?

Notes on chemicals

Acetic acid	Used in acid rinses (vinegar rinse).
Acetone	Solvent for nail enamel. Nail enamel remover (now rarely used).
Alkanolamide (alkylolamide)	Foam stabiliser in soapless shampoos.
Almond oil	Vegetable oil used for hot oil scalp treatments. Ingredient of control creams.
Ambergris	Secretion of sperm whale used in perfume to fix the odour.
Ammonium carbonate	Used as a catalyst to speed the release of oxygen from hydrogen peroxide during bleaching.
Ammonium hydroxide	An alkali used as a wetting agent and swelling agent in bleaches, perm lotions and tints to assist the penetration of other chemicals into the hair shaft. Active ingredient in heat perm lotions. Acts as a catalyst to speed the release of oxygen from hydrogen peroxide during bleaching.
Ammonium lauryl sulphate	A thick amber coloured liquid. A soapless detergent used in shampoos.
Ammonium thioglycollate (ammonium thiolethanoate)	A reducing agent. The active ingredient in cold wave lotion.
Amyl acetate	Solvent for nail enamel.
Apigenin	Active agent in camomile vegetable dyes.
Ascorbic acid (vitamin C)	A reducing agent and acid used to stop the action of hydrogen peroxide and to improve hair condition on completion of bleaching or tinting.
Borax (sodium borate)	Added to lacquer-removing shampoos.
Calamine (zinc carbonate)	Applied as lotion to skin irritation due to positive reaction to dye sensitivity test.
Calcium carbonate (limestone)	Deposited as fur or scale in kettles, etc., when temporary hard water is boiled.
Calcium bicarbonate	Causes temporary hardness in water.
Calcium oxide (quicklime)	Used in exothermic pads for heat perming.
Calcium stearate	Lime soap (scum) formed when soap is used in hard water.
Calcium sulphate	Causes permanent hardness in water.
Calgon (sodium hexametaphosphate)	Sequestering agent water softener sometimes added to shampoos or used as a rinse.
Camomile	Vegetable dye gives yellow cast to hair.
Carbaryl	Insecticide used to destroy head lice.
Carbon tetrachloride	Formerly used as wig cleaner.
Carbopol	Gelling agent for gel bleaches.

Carnauba wax	Obtained from surface of palm leaves. Ingredient of brilliantines.
Castor	Secretion from beavers used in perfumes to fix the odour.
Castor oil	Vegetable oil used in control creams and in manufacture of soap and soapless detergents.
Cetrimide (cetyl trimethyl ammonium bromide)	A quaternary ammonium compound. Cationic detergent and antiseptic which is substantive to hair. Used as conditioning and medicated shampoo. Added to many hairdressing products as a conditioner.
Cetyl alcohol	Emulsifying agent in conditioning creams and cream oxidation dyes.
Chlorofluoromethane	Volatile liquid used as aerosol propellant.
Citric acid	Acid rinse (lemon). Added to soapless shampoo as a conditioner.
Civet	Secretion from civet cat used in perfumes to fix the odour.
Coconut imidazoline	Soapless detergent for very mild shampoos.
Coconut oil	Vegetable oil used in manufacture of soap and soapless shampoos.
Collodion	Film-former to cover dye area in sensitivity test.
Cysteine	Amino acid formed by reduction of cystine during cold waving.
Cystine	Amino acid in keratin forming a linkage between adjacent polypeptide chains and containing a disulphide bond.
Diaminophenol (para-phenylenediamine)	Permanent oxidation dye (black).
Diaminotoluene (para-toluenediamine)	Permanent oxidation dye (brown).
Dimethyl hydantoin formaldehyde	Plastic resin film-former in lacquer and setting lotion.
Essential oils	Sweet smelling volatile plant oils used as perfumes. Some are mildly antiseptic.
Ethanol	Solvent for resins in lacquer and setting lotion.
Formaldehyde	Disinfectant gas produced by heating formalin.
Formalin (methanal)	Preservative for gum setting lotions and shampoos. Disinfectant liquid.
Glycerol	By-product of soap making. Used in hand creams and as a plasticiser in lacquers.

Glyceryl monothioglycollate	Reducing agent in acid perms.
Griseofulvin	Drug used to treat cases of ringworm.
Gum karaya	Gum for setting lotions.
Gum tragacanth	Gum for setting lotions.
Henna	Permanent vegetable dye (red shades).
Hexachlorophane	Antiseptic for medicated shampoos.
Hydrogen peroxide	An oxidising agent in bleaches, perm neutralisers and for oxidation of para dyes.
Isopropanol	Solvent for resin in lacquer and setting lotion. Cleaning mirrors.
Isopropyl myristate	Plasticiser in hair lacquer.
Lanette wax	Synthetic wax (mixture of cetyl and stearyl alcohols) used as an emulsifying agent in cosmetic creams.
Lanolin	Similar to sebum but obtained from sheep's wool. Conditioner in shampoos and plasticiser in lacquer.
Lanthionine	Amino acid formed during heat perming.
Lawsone	Active ingredient in henna dyes.
Liquid paraffin	Mineral oil used in control creams.
Lavender oil	Essential oil used in perfumes.
Lauryl diethanolamide	Foam stabiliser in soap and soapless shampoos.
Magnesium bicarbonate	Causes temporary hardness in water.
Magnesium carbonate (white henna)	White powder used as thickener in paste bleach.
Magnesium sulphate	Cause of permanent hardness in water.
Malathion	Insecticide used to destroy head lice.
Methylated spirit	Solvent for resin in lacquer and setting lotion.
Musk	Secretion from musk deer used to fix odour in perfumes.
Nitro-phenylenediamine (nitro-diaminobenzene)	Semi-permanent dye.
Oil of bay	Antiseptic essential oil used in medicated shampoo.
Olive oil	Vegetable oil used in making soap and soapless detergents. Hot oil treatments.
Paraffin oil	Mineral oil used in control creams.
Paraffin wax	Mineral wax used in control creams.
Para-hydroxyazobenzene	Azo dye produces temporary colour.
Para-phenylenediamine	Permanent oxidation dye.
Para-toluenediamine	Permanent oxidation dye.
Petroleum jelly (Vaseline)	Used to protect scalp during hair straightening by sodium hydroxide. Ingredient of solid brilliantine.

Phosphoric acid	Stabiliser for hydrogen peroxide added during manufacture.
Polyvinyl acetate	Plastic resin film-former for lacquer and setting lotion.
Polyvinyl pyrrolidone	Plastic resin film-former for lacquer and setting lotion. Substantive conditioner added to shampoos and perm lotions.
Protein hydrolysates	Substantive conditioners used in pre-perm fillers, perm lotions and shampoos.
Potassium hydroxide	Alkali used in making soft soap.
Potassium oleate	A soft soap used for shampoos.
Potassium persulphate	Oxidising agent added to bleaches as a booster.
Quaternary ammonium compounds	Antiseptics and conditioners (see cetrimide).
Salicylic acid	Stabiliser for hydrogen peroxide added during manufacture.
Selenium sulphide	Active ingredient in anti-dandruff shampoos.
Shellac	Natural resin used as film-former in lacquer.
Silicone oils	Provide water-resistant film in barrier creams, lacquers and setting lotions.
Silver nitrate	A salt used in metallic dyes.
Sodium bisulphite	Reducing agent used in heat perms.
Sodium bromate	Oxidising agent in perm neutralisers.
Sodium chloride (common salt)	Regenerates sodium ion exchange resin in water softeners. Thickener in soapless shampoos.
Sodium hexametaphosphate	See Calgon.
Sodium hydroxide (caustic soda)	Alkali used in manufacture of soap and soapless detergents. Active ingredient of some hair straighteners.
Sodium lauryl ether sulphate	Detergent used in clear soapless shampoos.
Sodium lauryl sulphate	Detergent used in cream soapless shampoos.
Sodium lauryl sarcosinate	Soapless detergent used in aerosol shampoos.
Sodium stearate	A hard soap.
Sodium sulphide	Used in two-application metallic dyes. Also a depilatory.
Spermaceti wax	Obtained from whales and used in control creams.
Stearic acid	Used in making soap and control creams.
Sulphonated castor oil (Turkey red oil)	Acts as both detergent and oil in conditioning shampoos.

Sulphonated olive oil	Acts as both detergent and oil in conditioning shampoos.
Sulphuric acid	Used in making soapless detergents.
Tartaric acid	Added to temporary acid dyes to make the dye cling to the hair.
Thioglycollic acid	Used in manufacture of perm lotion.
Trichlorethylene	Grease solvent used in wig cleaning.
Trichloroethane	Grease solvent used in wig cleaning.
Triethanolamine	An alkali used in making soaps and soapless detergents.
Triethanolamine lauryl sulphate	Detergent used in clear liquid soapless shampoos.
Turkey red oil	See sulphonated castor oil.
Vaseline	See petroleum jelly.
Witch hazel	An astringent in after shave lotion.
Zeolite	A natural resin formerly used in water softeners.
Zinc carbonate	See calamine.
Zinc pyrithione (zinc omadine)	Active ingredient in anti-dandruff shampoos.

Multiple choice questions

In the following questions, choose, in each case, the most suitable answer from the four possible alternatives given.

Chapter 1

1 Scalp hair is mostly
   (a) lanugo hair
   (b) fine hair
   (c) terminal hair
   (d) vellus hair

2 The name of the pigment in hair is
   (a) keratin
   (b) melanin
   (c) medulla
   (d) matrix

3 The protein of hair can be broken down into
   (a) amino acids
   (b) keratin
   (c) cytoplasm
   (d) acetic acid

4 The layers of a hair named from the outside to the centre are
   (a) cuticle, medulla, cortex
   (b) cortex, cuticle, medulla
   (c) medulla, cortex, cuticle
   (d) cuticle, cortex, medulla

5 A hygroscopic substance is one which
   (a) stretches when treated with water
   (b) contains a large proportion of water
   (c) absorbs moisture from the air
   (d) contains hydrogen atoms

6 Keratin is a chemical compound because it contains
   (a) a mixture of several different elements
   (b) several elements chemically united together
   (c) a mixture of atoms and molecules
   (d) a matrix of twisted fibres

7 The pH value of a neutral solution is
   (a) 1
   (b) 5
   (c) 7
   (d) 14

8 Traces of alkaline substances left on the hair after treatment may be neutralised by rinsing with
   (a) water
   (b) a salt solution
   (c) dilute acetic acid
   (d) concentrated sulphuric acid

9 The cuticle of a hair may be
damaged by

(a) backcombing
(b) dilute acids
(c) the application of lacquer
(d) steam treatment

10 The porosity of hair is decreased
by treatment with

(a) conditioning cream
(b) steam
(c) mild alkalis
(d) hot water

11 'Chemical neutralisation' results
in the formation of

(a) acids and alkalis
(b) acids and water
(c) salts and acids
(d) salts and water

12 Cystine is

(a) an alkali
(b) a polypeptide
(c) a salt
(d) an amino acid

13 Most of the pigment of hair
is situated in the

(a) medulla
(b) hair root
(c) cortex
(d) cuticle

14 Treatment with strong alkalis would
cause hair to

(a) become smoother
(b) disintegrate
(c) stretch
(d) become more hygroscopic

15 Organic compounds always contain
the element

(a) oxygen
(b) carbon
(c) sulphur
(d) nitrogen

16 Which one of the following
is not a salt?

(a) sodium stearate
(b) sodium chloride
(c) ammonium thioglycollate
(d) ammonium hydroxide

Chapter 2

1. The cells in the lowest layer of the
epidermis are

(a) constantly dividing
(b) made of keratin
(c) being constantly rubbed away
(d) flat and scaly

2 The horny layer of the epidermis

(a) secretes sebum
(b) forms a protective coat for the
body
(c) determines the colour of the
skin
(d) is an actively growing layer

3 The secretion from the sebaceous
glands

(a) cools the skin by evaporation
(b) removes waste products from
the skin
(c) lubricates the skin and hair
shaft
(d) nourishes the hair

4 A hair follicle is in the anagen stage of
its cycle when it is

(a) resting
(b) actively growing
(c) breaking down
(d) growing shorter

5 A hair grows from

(a) the inner root sheath
(b) the epidermal cells surrounding
the papilla
(c) the papilla itself
(d) the dermis

6 Contraction of the arrector pili
muscle causes a hair to

(a) stretch
(b) lie close to the head
(c) grow more quickly
(d) stand upright

7 Frequent cutting of the hair

(a) makes it grow faster
(b) slows the growth rate
(c) has no effect on growth rate
(d) makes it grow thicker

8 Elastic fibres in the skin are found
mainly in the

(a) dermis
(b) epidermis
(c) subcutaneous layer
(d) the hair follicles

9 The catagen stage in the growth cycle of a scalp hair lasts about

(a) 2 days
(b) 2 weeks
(c) 2 months
(d) 2 years

10 Exposure to ultra-violet rays causes

(a) kwashiorkor
(b) slowing of hair growth
(c) increased secretion of sweat
(d) increased melanin production

11 The germinating layer of the epidermis is also called the
(a) stratum lucidum
(b) stratum corneum
(c) basal layer
(d) granular layer

12 Skin pigment is produced by cells called

(a) pheomelanin
(b) melanocytes
(c) cytoplasm
(d) keratin

13 The secretion from the sweat glands consists mainly of

(a) sodium chloride
(b) sebum
(c) water
(d) oil

14 The secretion from the glands in the skin is

(a) slightly acid
(b) slightly alkaline
(c) strongly alkaline
(d) neutral

15 Huxley's layer is part of

(a) the dermis
(b) the inner root sheath
(c) the outer root sheath
(d) a hair shaft

16 The nerve endings of the skin are most frequently found in the

(a) epidermis
(b) dermis
(c) hair follicles
(d) hair papillae

Chapter 3

1 Proteins are mainly used by the body for

(a) the building of new tissue
(b) giving energy
(c) regulating body processes
(d) protecting the eyes

2 During digestion, protein foods are converted to

(a) glucose
(b) fatty acids
(c) amino acids
(d) carbohydrates

3 A growing hair is nourished by

(a) the germinating layer of the epidermis
(b) the application of conditioning cream
(c) nutrients from the blood vessels of the dermis
(d) sebum from the sebaceous glands

4 Iron is required in the diet to

(a) build strong teeth and bones
(b) make haemoglobin
(c) provide insulation
(d) prevent scurvy

5 Blood travels to the head by the

(a) pulmonary artery
(b) jugular vein
(c) carotid artery
(d) vena cava

6 The function of red blood cells is to

(a) fight bacteria
(b) help to secrete waste products
(c) carry oxygen round the body
(d) help in the clotting of blood

7 The smallest blood vessels are known as

(a) veins
(b) arteries
(c) plasma
(d) capillaries

8 The function of oxygen in the body is to

(a) enable breathing to take place
(b) oxidise sugar to produce energy
(c) improve the circulation of the blood
(d) build new body tissues

9 Arteries are blood vessels which carry

(a) only oxygenated blood
(b) only de-oxygenated blood
(c) blood to the heart
(d) blood away from the heart

10 The main artery of the body is called the

(a) aorta
(b) atrium
(c) carotid artery
(d) vena cava

11 Inhalation is caused by the

(a) contraction of muscles in the lungs
(b) relaxation of muscles in the lungs
(c) contraction of the muscles of the diaphragm and ribs
(d) relaxation of the muscles of the diaphragm and ribs

12 During internal respiration, glucose is oxidised to produce

(a) vitamin B
(b) energy
(c) oxygen
(d) enzymes

13 Glucose is a

(a) fat
(b) protein
(c) sugar
(d) starch

14 The digestion of protein starts in the

(a) mouth
(b) stomach
(c) small intestine
(d) large intestine

15 The digestion of all food is completed in the

(a) stomach
(b) small intestine
(c) large intestine
(d) rectum

16 Which of the following gases is present in air in the greatest proportion?

(a) nitrogen
(b) oxygen
(c) carbon dioxide
(d) hydrogen

Chapter 4

1 The epicranial aponeurosis is a

(a) muscle in the head
(b) bone in the skull
(c) vessel taking blood to the head
(d) sheet of tendon in the scalp

2 The lower jaw is known also as the

(a) maxilla
(b) mandible
(c) malar
(d) zygomatic

3 The parietal bones form the

(a) top of the cranium
(b) base of the cranium
(c) back of the skull
(d) sides of the skull

4 The saw-edged joints in the skull are called

(a) squamous
(b) sutures
(c) fontanelles
(d) strictures

5 'Orbit' is the name given to

(a) the external opening of the ear
(b) the eye ball
(c) the eye socket
(d) a bone at the base of the skull

6 The orbicularis oculi muscle

(a) closes the mouth
(b) moves the eye balls
(c) causes frowning
(d) closes the eye lids

7 The scalp may be moved by the

(a) occipito-frontalis muscle
(b) orbicularis oris
(c) temporalis and masseter
(d) orbicularis oculi

8 The bone forming the forehead is the

(a) temporal bone
(b) sphenoid bone
(c) frontal bone
(d) zygomatic bone

9 The part of the skull which protects the brain is called

(a) a suture
(b) the epicranial aponeurosis
(c) the orbit
(d) the cranium

10 The only movable bone in the skull is the

(a) ethmoid bone
(b) zygomatic arch
(c) lower jaw
(d) upper jaw

11 Which of the following are muscles of mastication?

(a) occipito-frontalis
(b) orbicularis oculi
(c) masseter and temporalis
(d) masseter and trapezius

12 The number of bones forming the cranium is

(a) 7
(b) 8
(c) 14
(d) 22

13 The thin sheet of muscle lying just below the skin in front of the neck is the

(a) sterno-mastoid
(b) trapezius
(c) temporalis
(d) platysma

14 The cranial bone through which the spinal cord passes is the

(a) sphenoid bone
(b) frontal bone
(c) occipital bone
(d) ethmoid bone

15 The shape of the tip of the nose is determined by

(a) a piece of cartilage
(b) a sheet of tendon
(c) the nasal bones
(d) the muscles of the nostrils

16 The zygomatic arch joins the

(a) temporal and sphenoid bones
(b) cheek bone and temporal bone
(c) cheek bone and sphenoid bone
(d) temporal and parietal bones

Chapter 5

1 A convex mirror produces an image which is

(a) magnified
(b) inverted
(c) smaller than the object
(d) equal in size to the object

2 A white matt surface

(a) reflects light in all directions
(b) reflects light in one direction only
(c) absorbs all the light
(d) refracts all the light

3 Two plane mirrors facing each other on the opposite sides of a corridor make it appear to be

(a) exactly half as wide
(b) exactly twice as high
(c) exactly twice as wide
(d) more than twice as wide

4 When a beam of light changes direction on passing into glass from the air it is being

(a) reflected
(b) refracted
(c) magnified
(d) intensified

5 Lacquer can be cleaned from mirrors by using

(a) carbon tetrachloride
(b) soap and water
(c) glycerol
(d) methylated spirit

6 A person 'sees' an object because

(a) light travels from the person's eyes to the object
(b) light travels from the object to the person's eyes
(c) the eyes reflect the light
(d) the sun shines on the object

7 A plane mirror placed along the length of one wall of a salon makes the salon appear

(a) exactly twice as large
(b) slightly larger
(c) slightly smaller
(d) half as big

8 When an object is placed between two mirrors which form a right angle, the number of images produced is

(a) 1   (c) 3
(b) 2   (d) 4

9   The rough surface of a hair causes light falling on it to be

  (a)   refracted
  (b)   diffused
  (c)   intensified
  (d)   absorbed

10   In a concave mirror the reflecting surface is

  (a)   perfectly flat
  (b)   on the inside of a curve
  (c)   on the outside of a curve
  (d)   on both sides of a curve

11   An object is opaque if

  (a)   no light is reflected from it
  (b)   no light passes through it
  (c)   the light passing through is diffused
  (d)   objects seen through it appear blurred

12   Glare may be caused by

  (a)   subdued lighting
  (b)   diffused lighting
  (c)   the reflection of bright light
  (d)   use of artificial light in day-time

13   If a concave mirror is held close to a person's face, the facial image is

  (a)   inverted
  (b)   magnified
  (c)   equal in size to the face
  (d)   reduced in size

14   Lateral inversion means that the image in a mirror appears

  (a)   inverted and diminished
  (b)   erect and enlarged
  (c)   slightly blurred at the edges
  (d)   to have its left and right sides interchanged

15   Glass is translucent, if light passing through it is

  (a)   reflected regularly
  (b)   refracted regularly
  (c)   refracted and diffused
  (d)   reflected and diffused

16   In a plane mirror the image is

  (a)   in front of the mirror
  (b)   as far behind the mirror as the object is in front
  (c)   twice as far behind the mirror as the object is in front
  (d)   smaller than the object

Chapter 6

1   A volatile substance is one which

  (a)   is used to treat fainting
  (b)   expands rapidly on heating
  (c)   has a high melting point
  (d)   evaporates quickly at room temperature

2   The molecules in a gas are

  (a)   vibrating about a fixed point
  (b)   larger than those in a liquid and move more slowly
  (c)   closely packed and move very slowly
  (d)   widely spaced and move rapidly

3   Condensation may occur in a salon if

  (a)   cold moist air meets a warm surface
  (b)   warm moist air meets a cold surface
  (c)   the humidity is too low
  (d)   the temperature is too high

4   Heat travels from the sun by

  (a)   conduction only
  (b)   radiation only
  (c)   radiation and conduction
  (d)   radiation and convection

5   The most comfortable type of under-clothing for wear in hot weather is made of

  (a)   cotton
  (b)   nylon
  (c)   rayon
  (d)   wool

6   Which of the following would be a suitable room temperature for a salon?

  (a)   20°C
  (b)   65°C
  (c)   70°C
  (d)   100°C

7   Water cooled from 4°C to 0°C

  (a)   condenses
  (b)   contracts
  (c)   expands
  (d)   melts

8   The air in a salon is often excessively humid due to

  (a)   the use of too many heaters
  (b)   air entering the salon from outside
  (c)   evaporation of moisture when drying hair
  (d)   the impurity of the air

9 Evaporation means the change of state from a

(a) liquid to a gas
(b) gas to a liquid
(c) liquid to a solid
(d) solid to a liquid

10 Normal body temperature is

(a) 20·0°C
(b) 32·0°C
(c) 36·9°C
(d) 98·4°C

11 When the human body is becoming over-heated

(a) the blood vessels in the skin dilate
(b) the blood vessels in the skin are constricted
(c) the secretion of perspiration decreases
(d) the arrector pili muscles contract

12 Which one of the following is a good conductor of heat?

(a) wood
(b) copper
(c) hair
(d) plastic

13 Compared with the air intake, the air breathed out contains a greater proportion of

(a) nitrogen
(b) oxygen
(c) carbon dioxide
(d) carbon monoxide

14 The main reason for discomfort in a badly ventilated salon is

(a) lacquer fumes
(b) excess carbon dioxide
(c) lack of oxygen
(d) high humidity

15 A hair hygrometer may be used to measure the

(a) the relative humidity of the air
(b) the moisture content of hair
(c) the thickness of hair
(d) the elasticity of hair

16 Which of the following is a chemical change?

(a) burning a fuel
(b) expansion of a metal
(c) rise in temperature of a substance
(d) water changing to steam

Chapter 7

1 A short circuit may be caused by

(a) faulty insulation
(b) overloading a circuit
(c) a blown fuse
(d) a faulty earth wire

2 An earth wire

(a) normally carries no current
(b) prevents the overloading of appliances
(c) controls the amount of current
(d) reduces the consumption of electricity

3 A domestic electricity meter measures the consumption of electricity in units called

(a) kilowatts
(b) kilowatt hours
(c) therms
(d) watts

4 Too many appliances plugged into one socket may

(a) cause a short circuit
(b) damage the appliances
(c) overload the circuit
(d) cause an electric shock

5 A plug may become hot due to

(a) a faulty connection
(b) a broken earth wire
(c) a blown main fuse
(d) too low a voltage

6 The insulation on the live wire of an appliance should be coloured

(a) black
(b) blue
(c) brown
(d) green and yellow

7 The maximum wattage of an appliance to be fitted with a 3 amp fuse on a supply with a mains voltage of 240 volts is

(a) 40
(b) 80
(c) 360
(d) 720

8 If electricity costs 5p a unit, what would be the total cost of using a 1500 watt hair dryer for 6 hours a day for five days?

(a) 45p
(b) 60p
(c) 120p
(d) 225p

9 Which of the following are often included in modern electrical installations instead of fuses?

(a) earth wires
(b) circuit breakers
(c) consumer units
(d) ring main circuits

10 The heating element of a radiant electric fire is made of

(a) copper wire
(b) nichrome
(c) tungsten
(d) aluminium

11 For how long could an appliance of 250 watts be used before consuming one unit of electricity?

(a) 1 hour
(b) 2 hours
(c) 3 hours
(d) 4 hours

12 The normal voltage of a domestic electricity supply in this country is

(a) 12 V
(b) 110 V
(c) 240 V
(d) 11 000 V

13 Electrical resistance is measured in

(a) volts
(b) amps
(c) watts
(d) ohms

14 Which of the following is the best electrical conductor?

(a) copper wire
(b) wet hair
(c) a damp comb
(d) the filament of a light bulb

15 A 9 kilowatt instantaneous water-heater should be fitted with a fuse of

(a) 5 A
(b) 15 A
(c) 30 A
(d) 45 A

16 The negatively charged particles in an atom are called

(a) electrons
(b) protons
(c) ions
(d) electrolytes

Chapter 8

1 A red object

(a) reflects mostly red light
(b) absorbs all the red light
(c) absorbs all colours of light
(d) reflects white light

2 In blue light, a red object would appear

(a) black
(b) blue
(c) purple
(d) red

3 The correct size of fuse for a mains lighting circuit is

(a) 5 A
(b) 13 A
(c) 15 A
(d) 30 A

4 Which of the following colours of light has the shortest wavelength?

(a) blue
(b) green
(c) red
(d) yellow

5 The power of an electric lamp is measured in

(a) amps
(b) kilowatt hours
(c) volts
(d) watts

6 The filament of an electric lamp is made of

(a) copper
(b) nichrome
(c) nickel
(d) tungsten

7 The light produced by a filament lamp is

(a) bluish-green
(b) reddish-yellow
(c) pure white
(d) red only

8 The powder coating the inside of a fluorescent tube is

(a) tungsten
(b) mercury vapour
(c) phosphorous
(d) a phosphor

9 The invisible rays just beyond the red end of a spectrum are

(a) X-rays
(b) ultra-violet rays
(c) light rays
(d) infra-red rays

10 Light split up by a prism into a spectrum has been

(a) diffused
(b) reflected
(c) deflected
(d) dispersed

11 An object appears black if all the light rays falling on it are

(a) absorbed
(b) reflected
(c) diffused
(d) dispersed

12 The glass bulb of a filament lamp contains an inert gas such as

(a) oxygen
(b) hydrogen
(c) nitrogen
(d) chlorine

13 Light-coloured walls are more suitable in a salon than dark walls because they

(a) do not become dirty as quickly
(b) reflect more light
(c) absorb more light
(d) are more attractive

14 Which of the following gives a light most similar in colour to daylight?

(a) 'warm white' fluorescent tubes
(b) 'white' fluorescent tubes
(c) pearl filament lamps
(d) sodium vapour lamps

15 The earth wire in a lighting circuit is installed in order to earth

(a) the filaments of the lamps
(b) the metal caps of the bulbs
(c) any metal light fittings
(d) the circuit switch

16 If several filament lamps in a room are wired in parallel

(a) the failure of one lamp causes the others to go out
(b) the failure of one lamp does not affect the others
(c) the failure of one lamp makes the others less bright
(d) each lamp requires a separate fuse

Chapter 9

1 The purpose of the waterseal in the trap below a shampoo basin is to
(a) collect any hair which passes down the waste pipe
(b) trap any small articles which are accidentally dropped down the pipe
(c) keep the drain free from bacteria
(d) prevent unpleasant odours from entering the salon

2 A solution is saturated if
(a) no more solvent will dissolve
(b) it contains the maximum amount of water
(c) no more solute will dissolve
(d) it contains too much water

3 Boiling temporary hard water produces a 'fur' of
(a) calcium carbonate
(b) calcium bicarbonate
(c) sodium bicarbonate
(d) calcium phosphate

4 The charged particles which will conduct an electric current through certain solutions are
(a) atoms
(b) molecules
(c) ions
(d) electrodes

5 Which of the following diseases is carried by water?
(a) measles
(b) typhoid
(c) pneumonia
(d) rickets

6 Soft water
(a) is chemically pure water
(b) gives a poor lather with soap
(c) forms a scum with soapless shampoo
(d) is free from dissolved calcium salts

7 A solvent is
(a) a soluble substance
(b) a substance which will dissolve
(c) a liquid in which another substance will dissolve
(d) an insoluble substance

8 Cold water pipes should be lagged with a
(a) good heat insulator
(b) good conductor of heat
(c) good radiator of heat
(d) poor radiator of heat

9 Chlorination of a town's water supply is carried out in order to

(a)   destroy germs
(b)   remove suspended dirt particles
(c)   make the water more palatable
(d)   prevent tooth decay

10 Distillation involves the processes of

(a)   boiling and convection
(b)   boiling and condensation
(c)   conduction and condensation
(d)   evaporation and solidification

11 A solution which will carry an electric current is called

(a)   a saturated solution
(b)   a homogeneous mixture
(c)   an electrolyte
(d)   an electrode

12 The deposit which may form on hair after using a soap shampoo in hard water, consists of

(a)   sodium stearate
(b)   calcium stearate
(c)   calcium carbonate
(d)   sodium bicarbonate

13 Chemically pure water should be used in a steamer because it

(a)   boils quicker than tap water
(b)   produces more steam
(c)   deposits no salts on heating
(d)   retains the heat longer

14 Temporary hardness in water is caused by

(a)   calcium carbonate
(b)   magnesium carbonate
(c)   magnesium bicarbonate
(d)   magnesium sulphate

15 Hard water may be softened by adding

(a)   carbon tetrachloride
(b)   calcium stearate
(c)   ammonium thioglycollate
(d)   sodium hexametaphosphate

16 Which of the following is most free from dissolved substances?

(a)   tap water
(b)   rain water
(c)   sea water
(d)   river water

Chapter 10

1 Which of the following substances is formed as a by-product during the manufacture of soap?
(a)   calcium stearate
(b)   glycerol
(c)   lanolin
(d)   sodium stearate

2 When potassium hydroxide is boiled with vegetable oils, the product is
(a)   soft soap
(b)   hard soap
(c)   soapless detergent
(d)   spirit soap

3 The temperature of water for shampooing should be about
(a)   20°C
(b)   40°C
(c)   60°C
(d)   100°C

4 A vinegar rinse contains
(a)   amino acid
(b)   acetic acid
(c)   citric acid
(d)   nitric acid

5 Which of the following may be used as an antiseptic in a medicated shampoo?
(a)   sodium hexametaphosphate
(b)   hexachlorophane
(c)   formaldehyde
(d)   triethanolamine

6 Which of the following is an astringent used in after-shave lotions?
(a)   acetic acid
(b)   alcohol
(c)   cetrimide
(d)   glycerol

7 A 'scum' of calcium stearate may be deposited on the hair due to
(a)   the use of a soapless detergent
(b)   not washing the shampoo out sufficiently
(c)   the use of a dry powder shampoo
(d)   the use of soap with hard water

8 Soapless shampoos are often preferred to soap shampoos because they
(a)   are cheaper
(b)   are easy to apply
(c)   do not leave a scum with hard water
(d)   do not de-grease the hair as much

9 A cream soapless shampoo consists mainly of

   (a)   sodium stearate
   (b)   sodium carbonate
   (c)   sodium hexametaphosphate
   (d)   sodium lauryl sulphate

10 A shampoo cleans hair by

   (a)   dissolving grease
   (b)   increasing surface tension
   (c)   forming a lather
   (d)   emulsifying grease

11 Which of the following is a soap?

   (a)   ammonium lauryl sulphate
   (b)   ammonium hydroxide
   (c)   sodium chloride
   (d)   potassium oleate

12 Which of the following is a cationic detergent?

   (a)   sodium stearate
   (b)   sodium lauryl sulphate
   (c)   cetrimide
   (d)   borax

13 The active ingredient in an antidandruff shampoo may be

   (a)   zinc pyrithione
   (b)   sodium alginate
   (c)   sodium hydroxide
   (d)   citric acid

14 An emulsifying agent

   (a)   consists of drops of oil suspended in water
   (b)   is a type of paint
   (c)   consists of oil dissolved in water
   (d)   is used to stabilise an emulsion

15 An emollient is

   (a)   a skin softener
   (b)   a hair remover
   (c)   an antiseptic lotion
   (d)   an astringent lotion

16 Which of the following groups of oils are volatile?

   (a)   essential oils
   (b)   fixed oils
   (c)   mineral oils
   (d)   vegetable oils

Chapter 11

1 The coiled polypeptide chains in keratin consist of

   (a)   amino acids
   (b)   cystine
   (c)   hydrogen bonds
   (d)   salt bonds

2 When hair is stretched

   (a) α-keratin becomes β-keratin
   (b) β-keratin becomes α-keratin
   (c)   the cystine linkages are broken
   (d)   a cohesive set is produced

3 When gum tragacanth is mixed with water, it forms

   (a)   an emulsion
   (b)   a suspension
   (c)   a mucilage
   (d)   a lather

4 A cohesive set is destroyed by

   (a)   a hot atmosphere
   (b)   a dry atmosphere
   (c)   a humid atmosphere
   (d)   too much sebum

5 A cohesive set is produced by

   (a)   perming
   (b)   water waving
   (c)   marcel waving
   (d)   steaming

6 Plastic setting lotions often contain

   (a)   gum tragacanth
   (b)   polypeptides
   (c)   sodium alginate
   (d)   polyvinyl pyrrolidone

7 The statement that 'hair is hygroscopic' means that hair will

   (a)   stretch when wet
   (b)   absorb moisture from the air
   (c)   dry quickly when heated
   (d)   grow rapidly

8 The elasticity of hair is mainly due to

   (a)   cystine linkages
   (b)   keratin
   (c)   polypeptide chains
   (d)   peptide linkages

9 Over processed hair does not take a good set because

   (a)   the cuticle is damaged
   (b)   it lacks elasticity
   (c)   the hair is too porous
   (d)   a coating of sebum is lacking

10 Hair is most elastic when it is

   (a)   completely dry
   (b)   wet with warm water
   (c)   treated with steam
   (d)   treated with a strong alkali

11 The most numerous of the cross linkages in keratin are the

   (a)   salt bonds
   (b)   cystine linkages
   (c)   hydrogen bonds
   (d)   peptide linkages

12 A cystine linkage contains

   (a)   two sulphur atoms
   (b)   two molecules of cystine
   (c)   amino acids
   (d)   cystine and cysteine

13 Humidity may be measured by use of a

   (a)   hydrometer
   (b)   barometer
   (c)   thermometer
   (d)   hygrometer

14 The solvent used in a plastic setting lotion is often

   (a)   ethanol
   (b)   polyvinyl resin
   (c)   lanolin
   (d)   borax

15 The plasticiser in plastic setting lotion may be

   (a)   glycerol
   (b)   ethanol
   (c)   cetrimide
   (d)   polyvinyl acetate

16 Formalin may be added to gum setting lotions

   (a)   to strengthen the gum
   (b)   as a plasticiser
   (c)   as a mould inhibitor
   (d)   as a perfume

Chapter 12

1. A bimetallic strip bends whilst being heated, because one metal

   (a)   is stronger than the other
   (b)   conducts heat better than the other
   (c)   expands more than the other
   (d)   becomes hotter than the other

2 A bimetallic strip is used

   (a)   as a heating element
   (b)   in a two-way switch
   (c)   for the two filaments in strip lighting
   (d)   in a thermostat

3 Evaporation is speeded by

   (a)   high temperature and high humidity
   (b)   low temperature and high humidity
   (c)   high temperature and low humidity
   (d)   low temperature and low humidity

4 The rate at which a liquid evaporates depends on

   (a)   its surface area
   (b)   the volume of liquid
   (c)   the weight of liquid
   (d)   its surface tension

5 Hair control creams are

   (a)   dilute solutions
   (b)   emulsions
   (c)   solvents
   (d)   saturated solutions

6 Which of the following could be used as the solvent in a hair lacquer?

   (a)   glycerol
   (b)   industrial methylated spirit
   (c)   polyvinyl acetate
   (d)   shellac

7 Atmospheric pressure is measured by using a

   (a)   barometer
   (b)   hydrometer
   (c)   hygrometer
   (d)   thermometer

8 An essential oil is

   (a)   necessary in hairdressing
   (b)   obtained from the ground
   (c)   a volatile oil
   (d)   a conditioning oil

9 An electric motor is necessary in

(a) infra-red dryers
(b) steamers
(c) blow dryers
(d) sterilising cabinets

10 The production of static electricity in newly dried hair after a shampoo and set, may be reduced by

(a) brushing vigorously
(b) using a cetrimide rinse before setting
(c) using a soapless shampoo
(d) drying with an infra-red dryer

11 Lanolin is obtained from

(a) the ground
(b) sebum
(c) sheep's wool
(d) shellac

12 Control creams add lustre to hair by

(a) increasing the reflection of light
(b) increasing the diffusion of light
(c) covering the hair with a transparent film
(d) adding more colour to the hair

13 The mineral oil in a control cream may be

(a) castor oil
(b) paraffin oil
(c) olive oil
(d) Turkey red oil

14 Shellac is a

(a) type of gum
(b) an essential oil
(c) a natural resin
(d) a synthetic resin

15 A shampoo designed to remove shellac-based lacquer may contain

(a) borax
(b) glycerol
(c) cetrimide
(d) lanolin

16 The plasticiser added to plastic hair lacquer during manufacture, will

(a) act as a solvent for the plastic resin
(b) strengthen the resin
(c) make the resin more pliable
(d) prevent the solvent from evaporating too quickly

Chapter 13

1 When hydrogen peroxide is used for bleaching, ammonia is added to

(a) stabilise the hydrogen peroxide
(b) speed the release of oxygen
(c) oxidise the hydrogen peroxide
(d) act as an emulsifying agent

2 If hydrogen peroxide is stored in a warm place it decomposes into

(a) oxygen and hydrogen
(b) hydrogen and water
(c) oxygen and water
(d) water only

3 The term '0:880' ammonia refers to

(a) any strong solution of ammonia
(b) the weight of ammonia required
(c) the volume of water required
(d) the relative density of the ammonia

4 During bleaching, melanin is

(a) changed to a colourless compound by oxidation
(b) washed out of the hair
(c) neutralised by the bleach
(d) changed to a colourless compound by reduction

5 A peroxometer is used to measure

(a) a particular volume of hydrogen peroxide
(b) the weight of peroxide required
(c) the density of hydrogen peroxide
(d) the volume strength of hydrogen peroxide

6 A basic oxide dissolved in water will form

(a) an acid
(b) an alkali
(c) a neutral solution
(d) a salt

7 The relative density of a liquid is

(a) the strength of the liquid
(b) its weight compared with that of an equal volume of water
(c) the number of parts by which the liquid has been diluted
(d) the weight of the strongest solution

8 Which one of the following substances can be used to provide oxygen for bleaching?

(a) calcium oxide
(b) carbon dioxide
(c) potassium persulphate
(d) potassium stearate

9 The heat from infra-red lamps is transferred to the client's head mainly by

(a) conduction
(b) convection
(c) reflection
(d) radiation

10 The process of bleaching hair is one of chemical

(a) decomposition
(b) neutralisation
(c) reduction
(d) oxidation

11 20 vol hydrogen peroxide solution has the same strength as a solution of

(a) 3%
(b) 6%
(c) 9%
(d) 12%

12 During the manufacture of hydrogen peroxide, salicylic acid may be added to

(a) increase the volume strength
(b) act as a catalyst
(c) stabilise the peroxide
(d) to act as an oxidising agent

13 During bleaching, hydrogen peroxide acts as

(a) a wetting agent
(b) an oxidising agent
(c) a reducing agent
(d) an emulsifying agent

14 Breakage of the hair by over-bleaching is due to the splitting of

(a) cystine linkages
(b) hydrogen bonds
(c) polypeptide chains
(d) salt bonds

15 The term '20 volume' hydrogen peroxide means that

(a) 20 ml of the peroxide is required
(b) the hydrogen peroxide is a 20% solution
(c) 20 ml of the peroxide will provide 20 ml of oxygen
(d) 1 ml of the peroxide will provide 20 ml of oxygen

16 'White henna' refers to

(a) ammonium persulphate
(b) ammonium carbonate
(c) magnesium carbonate
(d) magnesium peroxide

Chapter 14

1 During permanent colouring, the dye molecules
(a) swell in the cortex
(b) join together to form larger molecules in the cortex
(c) are reduced to enable them to enter the cortex
(d) are trapped in the medulla

2 Permanent colours are made alkaline during manufacture because alkalis will
(a) oxidise the dye molecules
(b) stabilise the added hydrogen peroxide
(c) return the hair to its natural acid state
(d) open the cuticle scales of the hair

3 Which one of the following is a vegetable dye?
(a) calamine
(b) camomile
(c) pyrogallol
(d) white henna

4 Which of the following dyes are most likely to cause dermatitis?
(a) azo dyes
(b) metallic dyes
(c) para dyes
(d) vegetable dyes

5 Which of the following is a semi-permanent dye?
(a) para-toluenediamine
(b) nitro-phenylenediamine
(c) para-phenylenediamine
(d) hydroxyazobenzene

6 If the pigment in hair absorbs all wavelengths of light the hair is coloured
(a) white
(b) black
(c) brown
(d) blonde

7 A skin test for oxidation dyes should be given
(a) occasionally
(b) before the first application only
(c) before each application
(d) every year

8 Unwanted orange shades developed during hair colouring may be corrected by adding a little
(a) red   (c) yellow
(b) green   (d) blue

9 The active ingredient in henna is

(a) indigo
(b) lanolin
(c) apigenin
(d) lawsone

10 Which of the following is a permanent dye?

(a) camomile
(b) hydroxyazobenzene
(c) nitro-phenylenediamine
(d) para- toluenediamine

11 To avoid contact dermatitis when applying a permanent tint, a hairdresser should

(a) always have a skin test before each application
(b) apply a hand cream
(c) wear protective gloves
(d) wash her hands immediately after applying the dye

12 Hair may be tinted lighter than the natural colour if the strength of peroxide used with a para dye is

(a) 10 vol
(b) 20 vol
(c) 30 vol
(d) 60 vol

13 Which of the following is often used as an antioxidant after a permanent dye?

(a) salicylic acid
(b) ascorbic acid
(c) phosphoric acid
(d) amino acid

14 Unwanted oxidation dyes may be removed by use of

(a) sodium formaldehyde sulphoxalate
(b) polyvinyl pyrrolidone
(c) sodium hexametaphosphate
(d) para-toluenediamine

15 Colour matching is best carried out

(a) in natural daylight
(b) under diffused lighting
(c) under fluorescent lighting
(d) under filament lamps

16 A yellow pigment normally reflects

(a) yellow light and a little green and blue
(b) yellow light and a little orange and green
(c) yellow and red light
(d) pure yellow light only

Chapter 15

1 Which of the following substances may be used instead of hydrogen peroxide in 'neutralisers'?

(a) ammonium hydroxide
(b) ammonium thioglycollate
(c) sodium bromate
(d) sodium stearate

2 Thioglycollic acid may be neutralised by

(a) acetic acid
(b) ammonium thioglycollate
(c) sodium chloride
(d) ammonium hydroxide

3 During 'neutralising' after a cold perm,

(a) cystine is oxidised to cysteine
(b) cystine is reduced to cysteine
(c) cysteine is oxidised to cystine
(d) cysteine is reduced to cystine

4 Exothermic pads may contain

(a) quicklime
(b) Calgon
(c) caustic soda
(d) caustic potash

5 The pH value of a cold wave lotion must not be greater than

(a) 6·5
(b) 7
(c) 9·5
(d) 14

6 The active ingredient in a cold wave lotion is

(a) ammonium hydroxide
(b) ammonium thioglycollate
(c) cetrimide
(d) hydrogen peroxide

7 Exothermic means

(a) giving out heat
(b) taking in heat
(c) without heat
(d) the number of therms used

8 A depilatory is

(a) a skin softener
(b) an astringent
(c) a hair remover
(d) an antiseptic

9 Hair which has had no previous treatment is known as

(a) lanugo hair
(b) virgin hair
(c) vellus hair
(d) natural hair

10 The presence of sebum on hair makes it

(a) less porous
(b) more hygroscopic
(c) more elastic
(d) easier to perm

11 The active ingredient in some hair straighteners is

(a) sodium carbonate
(b) sodium bicarbonate
(c) sodium hydroxide
(d) sodium stearate

12 Sodium hydroxide is

(a) an astringent
(b) a grease solvent
(c) caustic to the skin
(d) a skin emollient

13 Ammonium thioglycollate is

(a) an oxidising agent
(b) an emulsifying agent
(c) a neutralising agent
(d) a reducing agent

14 The cross linkages broken during perming are

(a) peptide linkages
(b) cystine linkages
(c) hydrogen bonds
(d) salt bonds

15 In cold waving, the hair should be wound

(a) as loosely as possible
(b) without tension
(c) so that the hair is stretched slightly
(d) as tightly as possible

16 The lotion used for heat perms contains

(a) sodium chloride
(b) sodium bicarbonate
(c) sodium perborate
(d) sodium bisulphite

Chapter 16

1 A pathogen is

(a) any minute organism
(b) a laboratory where diseases are studied
(c) an infectious disease
(d) an organism which causes disease

2 Infestation by head lice may lead to secondary infection such as

(a) dandruff
(b) impetigo
(c) dermatitis
(d) alopecia

3 Ringworm is caused by

(a) a virus
(b) bacterial infection
(c) an animal parasite
(d) a fungus

4 Dandruff is also known as

(a) pediculosis
(b) pityriasis
(c) psoriasis
(d) alopecia

5 Conjunctivitis is

(a) a disease of the hair shaft
(b) an infestation
(c) an infection of the eye
(d) a fungus disease

6 Which one of the following is contagious?

(a) alopecia
(b) ringworm
(c) psoriasis
(d) fragilitas crinium

7 The term 'folliculitis' indicates

(a) beaded hair shafts
(b) hair with split ends
(c) infection of the hair follicles
(d) ringworm of the scalp

8 Some bacteria can survive high temperature by forming

(a) spores
(b) cysts
(c) ova
(d) pathogens

9 Traction alopecia may be caused by

  (a) over-vigorous brushing
  (b) harsh chemicals
  (c) bacterial infection
  (d) the use of depilatories

10 Pediculosis capitis is caused by

  (a) itch mites
  (b) staphylococci
  (c) head lice
  (d) fungal infection

11 Which one of the following is a bacterial infection?

  (a) rickets
  (b) impetigo
  (c) influenza
  (d) scurvy

12 Bacteria may damage body cells by producing

  (a) spores
  (b) fungi
  (c) cysts
  (d) toxins

13 In the body tissues, germs may be killed by

  (a) white blood cells
  (b) red blood cells
  (c) blood platelets
  (d) blood plasma

14 Under which of the following conditions will bacteria multiply most rapidly?

  (a) cold, dry and light
  (b) warm, dry and light
  (c) warm, moist and dark
  (d) cold, moist and dark

15 Itch mites burrow into the

  (a) hair follicles
  (b) hair shaft
  (c) sebaceous glands
  (d) epidermis

16 Ringworm is treated by use of

  (a) griseofulvin
  (b) salicylic acid
  (c) malathion
  (d) zinc pyrithione

Chapter 17

1 In a salon the risk of spreading AIDS is reduced by

  (a) not touching an AIDS patient
  (b) using a UV cabinet
  (c) sterilisation of tools
  (d) use of strong disinfectants

2 The blades of electrical clippers may be disinfected by

  (a) washing with hot water
  (b) drying with a hair dryer
  (c) use of an alcohol-wipe
  (d) placing the clippers in a mild antiseptic solution

3 In an ultra-violet sterilising cabinet, germs are killed by

  (a) a disinfectant gas
  (b) the effect of radiation
  (c) heat
  (d) dehydration

4 'Athlete's foot' would require treatment with a

  (a) deodorant
  (b) fungicide
  (c) disinfectant
  (d) bactericide

5 Influenza is caused by

  (a) a virus infection
  (b) a fungus
  (c) a bacteria infection
  (d) animal parasites

6 Psoriasis is

  (a) an infestation
  (b) a fungal disease
  (c) a non-infectious condition
  (d) a virus disease

7 Increasing the pressure on water which is being heated causes its

  (a) temperature to rise
  (b) temperature to decrease
  (c) boiling point to decrease
  (d) boiling point to increase

8 Ultra-violet rays

  (a) are damaging to the eyes
  (b) produce vitamin C in the skin
  (c) have a longer wavelength than infra-red rays
  (d) are used for high frequency treatments

9 Ringworm may be passed from one person to another by

   (a) inhaling infected air-borne droplets

   (b) contaminated water supplies

   (c) contact with an infected object

   (d) eating infected food

10 Athlete's foot may result from

   (a) excessive perspiration

   (b) lack of cleanliness

   (c) walking in an infected area

   (d) droplet infection

11 Sterilisation by boiling under increased pressure is called

   (a) autoclaving

   (b) distillation

   (c) de-ionisation

   (d) dehydration

12 Towels are best disinfected by

   (a) soaking before washing

   (b) boiling before washing

   (c) machine washing

   (d) treating with formaldehyde

13 The effectiveness of cetrimide is destroyed by

   (a) soap

   (b) alcohol

   (c) hot water

   (d) cold water

14 Sterilisation means

   (a) placing tools in a sterilising cabinet

   (b) complete destruction of living organisms

   (c) prevention of the spread of germs

   (d) using strong antiseptics

15 Sun-burn is caused by

   (a) X-rays

   (b) ultra-violet rays

   (c) infra-red rays

   (d) visible light rays

16 Which of the following may be used as an antiseptic?

   (a) formaldehyde

   (b) selenium sulphide

   (c) triethanolamine

   (d) cetrimide

Chapter 18

1 The main function of sweat is to

   (a) lubricate the skin

   (b) cool the skin

   (c) keep the skin moist

   (d) remove waste from the skin

2 Finger nails are composed of

   (a) bone tissue

   (b) cystine

   (c) keratin

   (d) cartilage

3 Finger nails grow from the

   (a) dermis

   (b) nail fold

   (c) lunula

   (d) germinal matrix

4 Ill-fitting shoes can cause

   (a) athlete's foot

   (b) plantar warts

   (c) corns

   (d) rickets

5 Muscles are attached to bones by

   (a) tendons

   (b) ligaments

   (c) cartilage

   (d) gristle

6 One function of vitamin C in the body is to

   (a) release energy from carbo-hydrates

   (b) build strong teeth and bones

   (c) build up the cementing material between cells

   (d) protect the eyes

7 Which of the following could be used as a plasticiser in nail lacquer?

   (a) plastic resin

   (b) amyl acetate

   (c) acetone

   (d) glycerol

8 Which of the following is a ball and socket joint?

   (a) the knee

   (b) the ankle

   (c) the hip

   (d) the elbow

9 Perspiration odour is associated with

(a) apocrine glands
(b) eccrine glands
(c) sebaceous glands
(d) endocrine glands

10 The term 'halitosis' refers to

(a) excessive perspiration
(b) tooth decay
(c) insensible perspiration
(d) unpleasant breath odours

11 The half moon at the base of a nail is also called the

(a) nail bed
(b) matrix
(c) lunula
(d) cuticle

12 The main body of a nail is the

(a) nail plate
(b) nail root
(c) germinal matrix
(d) nail fold

13 Which of the following is least likely to cause contact dermatitis?

(a) para dye
(b) soap shampoo
(c) soapless shampoo
(d) ammonium thioglycollate

14 Which of the following foods provides a good source of vitamin C?

(a) blackcurrants
(b) milk
(c) liver
(d) cereals

15 Which one of the following is not composed mainly of keratin?

(a) nails
(b) hair
(c) the horny layer of the epidermis
(d) the basal layer of the epidermis

16 Which of the following are involuntary muscles?

(a) muscles of facial expression
(b) heart muscles
(c) muscles of mastication
(d) muscles which move the arms

Chapter 19

1 If perm lotion has entered a client's eye,
(a) rinse the eye with plenty of water
(b) send for medical aid
(c) cover it with cotton wool
(d) rinse the eye with neutraliser

2 A cold compress would be useful on a
(a) boil
(b) chemical burn
(c) scald
(d) sprained ankle

3 Before commencing artificial respiration
(a) give the patient a cup of tea
(b) obtain medical aid
(c) place the patient in the recovery position
(d) ensure that the air passages are open

4 A sterile dressing is one which
(a) is completely germ free
(b) has just been washed
(c) has been treated with disinfectant
(d) contains a bandage and cotton wool

5 A minor burn on the hand should be treated by
(a) rubbing the area with cold cream
(b) bandaging tightly to keep the air out
(c) running cold water over the area
(d) applying antiseptic

6 Which of the following gases must be present if combustion is to take place?
(a) carbon dioxide
(b) carbon monoxide
(c) oxygen
(d) nitrogen

7 Which of the following is a flammable liquid used in hair lacquer aerosols?
(a) chlorofluoromethane
(b) carbon tetrachloride
(c) industrial methylated spirit
(d) plastic resin

8 If a person feels faint, they should
(a) lie completely flat
(b) place their head between their knees
(c) be wrapped in a blanket
(d) be taken to a doctor

9 Salon fire extinguishers sometimes contain compressed

   (a) oxygen
   (b) nitrogen
   (c) carbon monoxide
   (d) carbon dioxide

10 A chemical burn on the skin may be caused by contact with

   (a) citric acid solution
   (b) hot oil
   (c) 60 vol hydrogen peroxide
   (d) carbon tetrachloride

11 Diabetes is caused by lack of

   (a) vitamin C
   (b) insulin
   (c) haemoglobin
   (d) calcium

12 Hydrogen peroxide should not be stored near flammable chemicals because it

   (a) easily ignites
   (b) is a volatile liquid
   (c) assists fire
   (d) gives off hydrogen

13 Which one of the following is a non-corrosive poison?

   (a) aspirin
   (b) household bleach
   (c) strong ammonium hydroxide
   (d) caustic soda

14 Concussion may be caused by

   (a) shock following bad news
   (b) an electric shock
   (c) a blow to the head
   (d) a seizure

15 If a client suffers from a bleeding nose

   (a) place a cold key at the back of the neck
   (b) place the patient on the floor with the head lower than the feet
   (c) send for a doctor immediately
   (d) bend the head forwards and pinch the nostrils together

16 If a salon fire is out of control you should first

   (a) telephone the Fire Service
   (b) complete all hairdressing as quickly as possible
   (c) ensure that all clients and staff leave the building
   (d) open windows to allow the escape of smoke

Answers to Multiple Choice Questions

Chapter 1

Question	1	2	3	4	5	6	7	8	9	10	11	12	13	14	15	16
Answer	c	b	a	d	c	b	c	c	a	a	d	d	c	b	b	d

Chapter 2

Question	1	2	3	4	5	6	7	8	9	10	11	12	13	14	15	16
Answer	a	b	c	b	b	d	c	a	b	d	c	b	c	a	b	b

Chapter 3

Question	1	2	3	4	5	6	7	8	9	10	11	12	13	14	15	16
Answer	a	c	c	b	c	c	d	b	d	a	c	b	c	b	b	a

Chapter 4

Question	1	2	3	4	5	6	7	8	9	10	11	12	13	14	15	16
Answer	d	b	a	b	c	d	a	c	d	c	c	b	d	c	a	b

Chapter 5

Question	1	2	3	4	5	6	7	8	9	10	11	12	13	14	15	16
Answer	c	a	d	b	d	b	a	c	b	b	b	c	b	d	c	b

Chapter 6

Question	1	2	3	4	5	6	7	8	9	10	11	12	13	14	15	16
Answer	d	d	b	b	a	a	c	c	a	c	a	b	c	d	a	a

Chapter 7

Question	1	2	3	4	5	6	7	8	9	10	11	12	13	14	15	16
Answer	a	a	b	c	a	c	d	d	b	b	d	c	d	a	d	a

Chapter 8

Question	1	2	3	4	5	6	7	8	9	10	11	12	13	14	15	16
Answer	a	a	a	a	d	d	b	d	d	d	a	c	b	a	c	b

Chapter 9

Question	1	2	3	4	5	6	7	8	9	10	11	12	13	14	15	16
Answer	d	c	a	c	b	d	c	a	a	b	c	b	c	c	d	b

Chapter 10

Question	1	2	3	4	5	6	7	8	9	10	11	12	13	14	15	16
Answer	b	a	b	b	b	b	b	d	c	d	d	d	c	a	d	a	a

Chapter 11

Question	1	2	3	4	5	6	7	8	9	10	11	12	13	14	15	16
Answer	a	a	c	c	b	d	b	c	b	c	c	a	d	a	a	c

Chapter 12

Question	1	2	3	4	5	6	7	8	9	10	11	12	13	14	15	16
Answer	c	d	c	a	b	b	a	c	c	b	c	a	b	c	a	c

Chapter 13

Question	1	2	3	4	5	6	7	8	9	10	11	12	13	14	15	16
Answer	b	c	d	a	d	b	b	c	d	d	b	c	b	c	d	c

Chapter 14

Question	1	2	3	4	5	6	7	8	9	10	11	12	13	14	15	16
Answer	b	d	b	c	b	b	c	d	d	d	c	c	b	a	a	b

Chapter 15

Question	1	2	3	4	5	6	7	8	9	10	11	12	13	14	15	16
Answer	c	d	c	a	c	b	a	c	b	a	c	c	d	b	b	d

Chapter 16

Question	1	2	3	4	5	6	7	8	9	10	11	12	13	14	15	16
Answer	d	b	d	b	c	b	c	a	a	c	b	d	a	c	d	a

Chapter 17

Question	1	2	3	4	5	6	7	8	9	10	11	12	13	14	15	16
Answer	c	c	b	b	a	c	d	a	c	c	a	b	a	b	b	d

Chapter 18

Question	1	2	3	4	5	6	7	8	9	10	11	12	13	14	15	16
Answer	b	c	d	c	a	c	d	c	a	d	c	a	b	a	d	b

Chapter 19

Question	1	2	3	4	5	6	7	8	9	10	11	12	13	14	15	16
Answer	a	d	d	a	c	c	c	b	d	c	b	c	a	c	d	c

Index

191